Clinical Examination

Editor

BRIAN T. GARIBALDI

MEDICAL CLINICS
OF NORTH AMERICA

www.medical.theclinics.com

Consulting Editor
BIMAL H. ASHAR

May 2018 • Volume 102 • Number 3

ELSEVIER

1600 John F. Kennedy Boulevard • Suite 1800 • Philadelphia, Pennsylvania, 19103-2899

http://www.theclinics.com

MEDICAL CLINICS OF NORTH AMERICA Volume 102, Number 3
May 2018 ISSN 0025-7125, ISBN-13: 978-0-323-58362-6

Editor: Jessica McCool
Developmental Editor: Kristen Helm

Medical Clinics of North America (ISSN 0025-7125) is published bimonthly by Elsevier Inc., 360 Park Avenue South, New York, NY 10010-1710. Months of publication are January, March, May, July, September, and November. Business and editorial offices: 1600 John F. Kennedy Boulevard, Suite 1800, Philadelphia, PA 19103-2899. Periodicals postage paid at New York, NY, and additional mailing offices. Subscription prices are USD $273.00 per year (US individuals), $574.00 per year (US institutions), $100.00 per year (US Students), $336.00 per year (Canadian individuals), $746.00 per year (Canadian institutions), $200.00 per year (Canadian and foreign students), $402.00 per year (foreign individuals), and $746.00 per year (foreign institutions). To receive student/resident rate, orders must be accompanied by name of affiliated institution, date of term, and the signature of program/residency coordinator on institution letterhead. Orders will be billed at individual rate until proof of status is received. Foreign air speed delivery is included in all Clinics' subscription prices. All prices are subject to change without notice. **POSTMASTER:** Send address changes to *Medical Clinics of North America*, Elsevier Health Sciences Division, Subscription Customer Service, 3251 Riverport Lane, Maryland Heights, MO 63043. **Customer Service: Telephone: 1-800-654-2452** (U.S. and Canada); **1-314-447-8871** (outside U.S. and Canada). **Fax: 314-447-8029. E-mail: journalscustomerserviceusa@elsevier.com** (for print support); **journalsonlinesupport-usa@elsevier.com** (for online support).

Reprints. For copies of 100 or more of articles in this publication, please contact the Commercial Reprints Department, Elsevier Inc., 360 Park Avenue South, New York, NY 10010-1710. Tel.: 212-633-3874; Fax: 212-633-3820; E-mail: reprints@elsevier.com.

Medical Clinics of North America is also published in Spanish by McGraw-Hill Interamericana Editores S. A., P.O. Box 5-237, 06500 Mexico, D.F., Mexico.

Medical Clinics of North America is covered in *MEDLINE/PubMed (Index Medicus), Current Contents, ASCA, Excerpta Medica, Science Citation Index,* and *ISI/BIOMED.*

PROGRAM OBJECTIVE
The goal of the *Medical Clinics of North America* is to keep practicing physicians up to date with current clinical practice by providing timely articles reviewing the state of the art in patient care.

TARGET AUDIENCE
All practicing physicians and other healthcare professionals.

LEARNING OBJECTIVES
Upon completion of this activity, participants will be able to:
1. Review the outpatient physical examination.
2. Discuss the clinical examination, diagnostic errors and the role of technology in the bedside encounter.
3. Recognize digital tools and improving observation skills to enhance the clinical examination.

ACCREDITATION
The Elsevier Office of Continuing Medical Education (EOCME) is accredited by the Accreditation Council for Continuing Medical Education (ACCME) to provide continuing medical education for physicians.

The EOCME designates this enduring material for a maximum of 15 *AMA PRA Category 1 Credit*(s)™. Physicians should claim only the credit commensurate with the extent of their participation in the activity.

All other healthcare professionals requesting continuing education credit for this enduring material will be issued a certificate of participation.

DISCLOSURE OF CONFLICTS OF INTEREST
The EOCME assesses conflict of interest with its instructors, faculty, planners, and other individuals who are in a position to control the content of CME activities. All relevant conflicts of interest that are identified are thoroughly vetted by EOCME for fair balance, scientific objectivity, and patient care recommendations. EOCME is committed to providing its learners with CME activities that promote improvements or quality in healthcare and not a specific proprietary business or a commercial interest.

The planning committee, staff, authors and editors listed below have identified no financial relationships or relationships to products or devices they or their spouse/life partner have with commercial interest related to the content of this CME activity:
Maja K. Artandi, MD; Bimal H. Ashar, MD, MBA, FACP; Hal H. Atkinson, MD; Alejandra Ellison-Barnes, MD; Jeff Chi, MD; Bennett W. Clark, MD; Lisa A. Cooper, MD, MPH; Cari Costanzo, PhD; Arsalan Derakhshan, MD; Sanjay V. Desai, MD; Gurpreet Dhaliwal, MD; Charles R. Doarn, MBA; Andrew Elder, BSc, MBCHB, FRCP, FRCPSG, FRCP(Edin), FACP, FICP(Hon); Brian T. Garibaldi, MD; Jeremy A. Greene, MD; Helene F. Hedian, MD; Erica N. Johnson, MD; Alison Kemp; Elizabeth A. Krupinski, PhD; John Kugler, MD; Andre Kumar, MD; Peter R. Lichstein, MD; Gigi Liu, MD; Reza Manesh, MD; Sherine Mathew, MD; Jessica McCool; Karly A. Murphy, MD; Timothy M. Niessen, MD; Andrew P.J. Olson, MD; Sharon Onguti, MD; Stephen W. Russell, MD; Rosalyn W. Stewart, MD, MS, MBA; Jeyanthi Surendrakumar; Christine Todd, MD; Abraham Verghese, MD, MACP, FRCP(Edin); Ronald S. Weinstein, MD; Junaid A.B. Zaman, MA, BMBCh, MRCP.

The planning committee, staff, authors and editors listed below have identified financial relationships or relationships to products or devices they or their spouse/life partner have with commercial interest related to the content of this CME activity:

UNAPPROVED/OFF-LABEL USE DISCLOSURE
The EOCME requires CME faculty to disclose to the participants:
1. When products or procedures being discussed are off-label, unlabelled, experimental, and/or investigational (not US Food and Drug Administration [FDA] approved); and
2. Any limitations on the information presented, such as data that are preliminary or that represent ongoing research, interim analyses, and/or unsupported opinions. Faculty may discuss information about pharmaceutical agents that is outside of FDA-approved labelling. This information is intended solely for CME and is not intended to promote off-label use of these medications. If you have any questions, contact the medical affairs department of the manufacturer for the most recent prescribing information.

TO ENROLL
To enroll in the *Medical Clinics of North America* Continuing Medical Education program, call customer service at 1-800-654-2452 or sign up online at http://www.theclinics.com/home/cme. The CME program is available to subscribers for an additional annual fee of USD $300.90.

METHOD OF PARTICIPATION

In order to claim credit, participants must complete the following:

1. Complete enrolment as indicated above.
2. Read the activity.
3. Complete the CME Test and Evaluation. Participants must achieve a score of 70% on the test. All CME Tests and Evaluations must be completed online.

CME INQUIRIES/SPECIAL NEEDS

For all CME inquiries or special needs, please contact elsevierCME@elsevier.com.

MEDICAL CLINICS OF NORTH AMERICA

ISSUE OF RELATED INTEREST

Clinics in Geriatric Medicine, August 2017 (Vol. 33, No. 3)
Rapid Geriatric Assessment
John E. Morley, *Editor*
Available at: http://www.geriatric.theclinics.com/

Contributors

CONSULTING EDITOR

BIMAL H. ASHAR, MD, MBA, FACP
Associate Professor of Medicine, Division of General Internal Medicine, Johns Hopkins University School of Medicine, Baltimore, Maryland, USA

EDITOR

BRIAN T. GARIBALDI, MD
Co-President, Society of Bedside Medicine, Assistant Professor of Medicine and Physiology, Division of Pulmonary and Critical Care, Johns Hopkins University School of Medicine, Baltimore, Maryland, USA

AUTHORS

MAJA K. ARTANDI, MD
Clinical Associate Professor, Department of Medicine, Stanford University, Palo Alto, California, USA

HAL H. ATKINSON, MD
Professor of Medicine, Department of Internal Medicine, Section on General Internal Medicine and Section on Gerontology and Geriatric Medicine, Wake Forest School of Medicine, Winston Salem, North Carolina, USA

JEFF CHI, MD
Clinical Associate Professor, Department of Medicine, Division of Hospital Medicine, Stanford University, Stanford, California, USA

BENNETT W. CLARK, MD
Department of Internal Medicine, University of Minnesota Medical School, Minneapolis, Minnesota, USA

LISA A. COOPER, MD, MPH
Bloomberg Distinguished Professor, James F. Fries Professor, Department of Medicine, Director, Johns Hopkins Center for Health Equity, Johns Hopkins University School of Medicine, Department of Health, Behavior and Society, Johns Hopkins Bloomberg School of Public Health, Center for Health Equity, Johns Hopkins University, Baltimore, Maryland, USA

CARI COSTANZO, PhD
Lecturer, Department of Anthropology, Undergraduate Advising and Research, Stanford University, Stanford, California, USA

ARSALAN DERAKHSHAN, MD
Department of Internal Medicine, Johns Hopkins University School of Medicine, Baltimore, Maryland, USA

SANJAY V. DESAI, MD
Department of Internal Medicine, Johns Hopkins University School of Medicine, Baltimore, Maryland, USA

GURPREET DHALIWAL, MD
Professor, Department of Medicine, University of California, San Francisco, Medical Service, San Francisco VA Medical Center, San Francisco, California, USA

CHARLES R. DOARN, MBA
Professor, Department of Family and Community Medicine, University of Cincinnati, Cincinnati, Ohio, USA

ANDREW ELDER, BSc, MBCHB, FRCP, FRCPSG, FRCP(Edin), FACP, FICP(Hon)
Honorary Professor and Consultant Physician, Professor, Department of Acute Medicine for Older People, Edinburgh Medical School, Western General Hospital, Edinburgh, United Kingdom

ALEJANDRA ELLISON-BARNES, MD
Osler Medical Residency Training Program, Department of Medicine, Johns Hopkins Hospital, Baltimore, Maryland, USA

BRIAN T. GARIBALDI, MD
Co-President, Society of Bedside Medicine, Assistant Professor of Medicine and Physiology, Division of Pulmonary and Critical Care, Johns Hopkins University School of Medicine, Baltimore, Maryland, USA

JEREMY A. GREENE, MD, PhD
Professor, Departments of Medicine and the History of Medicine, Johns Hopkins University School of Medicine, Baltimore, Maryland, USA

HELENE F. HEDIAN, MD
Assistant Professor, Division of General Internal Medicine, Johns Hopkins University School of Medicine, Baltimore, Maryland, USA

ERICA N. JOHNSON, MD
Program Director, Johns Hopkins Bayview Internal Medicine Residency, Assistant Professor, Department of Medicine, Division of Infectious Diseases, Johns Hopkins University School of Medicine, Johns Hopkins Bayview Medical Center, Baltimore, Maryland, USA

ELIZABETH A. KRUPINSKI, PhD
Professor and Vice Chair for Research, Department of Radiology and Medical Imaging, Emory University, Atlanta, Georgia, USA

JOHN KUGLER, MD
Clinical Associate Professor, Department of Medicine, Division of Hospital Medicine, Stanford University, Stanford, California, USA

ANDRE KUMAR, MD
Clinical Instructor, Department of Medicine, Division of Hospital Medicine, Stanford University, Stanford, California, USA

PETER R. LICHSTEIN, MD
Professor of Medicine, Department of Internal Medicine, Section on General Internal Medicine and Section on Gerontology and Geriatric Medicine, Wake Forest School of Medicine, Winston Salem, North Carolina, USA

GIGI LIU, MD, MSc
Instructor, Department of Medicine, Johns Hopkins University, Baltimore, Maryland, USA

REZA MANESH, MD
Assistant Professor, Department of Internal Medicine, Johns Hopkins Hospital, Johns Hopkins University School of Medicine, Baltimore, Maryland, USA

SHERINE MATHEW, MD
Internal Medicine Resident, Post Graduate Year One, Department of Internal Medicine, Southern Illinois University School of Medicine, Springfield, Illinois, USA

KARLY A. MURPHY, MD
General Internal Medicine Fellow, Department of Medicine, Johns Hopkins Hospital, Baltimore, Maryland, USA

TIMOTHY M. NIESSEN, MD, MPH
Assistant Professor, Division of General Internal Medicine, Hospitalist Program, Johns Hopkins University School of Medicine, Baltimore, Maryland, USA

ANDREW P.J. OLSON, MD
Assistant Professor of Medicine and Pediatrics, Divisions of General Internal Medicine and Hospital Pediatrics, University of Minnesota Medical School, Minneapolis, Minnesota, USA

SHARON ONGUTI, MD
Assistant Professor and Associate Clerkship Director, Department of Internal Medicine, Southern Illinois University School of Medicine, Springfield, Illinois, USA

STEPHEN W. RUSSELL, MD
Associate Professor of Internal Medicine and Pediatrics, Department of Medicine, University of Alabama, Birmingham, Alabama, USA; UAB Medicine-Leeds, Leeds, Alabama, USA

ROSALYN W. STEWART, MD, MS, MBA
Associate Professor, Departments of Medicine and Pediatrics, Johns Hopkins University, Baltimore, Maryland, USA

CHRISTINE TODD, MD
Assistant Professor and Chair, Department of Medical Humanities, Department of Internal Medicine, Southern Illinois University School of Medicine, Springfield, Illinois, USA

ABRAHAM VERGHESE, MD, MACP, FRCP(Edin)
Linda R. Meier and Joan F. Lane Provostial Professor, Vice Chair for the Theory and Practice of Medicine, Department of Medicine, Stanford University, Stanford, California, USA

RONALD S. WEINSTEIN, MD, FCAP
Founding Director, Arizona Telemedicine Program, Professor of Pathology, The University of Arizona College of Medicine, Tucson, Arizona, USA

JUNAID A.B. ZAMAN, MA, BMBCh, MRCP
Fulbright British Heart Foundation Scholar, Stanford University, Palo Alto, California, USA; Clinical Electrophysiology Fellow, Good Samaritan Hospital, Los Angeles, California, USA; Honorary Clinical Research Fellow, Imperial College London, London, United Kingdom

Contents

Technology has the potential to both distract and reconnect providers with their patients. The widespread adoption of electronic medical records in recent years pulls physicians away from time at the bedside. However, when used in conjunction with patients, technology has the potential to bring patients and physicians together. The increasing use of point-of-care ultrasound by physicians is changing the bedside encounter by allowing for real-time diagnosis with the treating physician. It is a powerful example of the way technology can be a force for refocusing on the bedside encounter.

Diagnostic errors are common in clinical practice and lead to adverse patient outcomes. Systematic reviews have shown that inadequate history taking and physical examination lead to a plurality, if not a majority, of diagnostic errors. Recent advances in cognitive science have also shown that unconscious biases likely contribute to many diagnostic errors. Research into diagnostic error has been hampered by methodologic inconsistency and a paucity of studies in real-world clinical settings. The best evidence indicates that educational interventions to reduce diagnostic error should give physicians feedback about clinical outcomes and enhance their ability to recognize signs and symptoms of specific diseases at the bedside.

The physical examination in the outpatient setting is a valuable tool. Even in settings where there is lack of evidence, such as the annual physical examination of an asymptomatic adult, the physical examination is beneficial for the physician-patient relationship. When a patient has specific symptoms, the physical examination, in addition to a thorough history, can help narrow down, or in many cases establish, a diagnosis. In a time where imaging and laboratory tests are easily available, but are expensive and can be invasive, a skilled physical examination remains an important component of patient evaluation.

This article examines how the adoption of the electronic health record (EHR) has changed the most fundamental unit of medicine: the clinical examination. The impact of the EHR on the clinical history, physical examination, documentation, and the doctor-patient relationship is described. The EHR now has a dominant role in clinical care and will be a central factor in clinical work of the future. Conversation needs to be shifted toward defining best practices with current EHRs inside and outside of the examination room.

At the heart of every effective patient-physician interaction is a relationship that is built on trust. Cultivating sound communication skills coupled with the awareness and application of ethical principles is integral to this process. One of the foremost challenges in competent practice is negotiating situations that arise at the bedside when such issues as patient autonomy, differing world views, honesty, and cost stewardship come into conflict. It is essential for health care providers to consider how to detect and prioritize these issues as they advocate for high-quality and patient-centered care.

For much of the twentieth century, educators lacked evidence that teaching observational skills could benefit modern medicine. But in 2001, a statistical model emerged that supported the effectiveness of teaching observational skills to medical students using a museum-based curriculum. The story that led to that ground-breaking study, and the consequences that sprung from it, is retold here, traveling from the darkened caves in the foothills of France to the brightly lit galleries of the Yale Center for British Art. It never would have happened without the indelible mark made by one curious man's journey.

Bedside hospital rounds promote patient-centered care in teaching and nonteaching settings. Patients and families prefer bedside rounds, and provider acceptance is increasing. Efficient bedside rounds with an interprofessional team or with learners requires preparation of the patient and the rounding team. Bedside "choreography" provides structure and sets expectations for time spent in the room. By using relationship-centered communication, rounds can be both patient proximate and patient centered. The clinical examination can be integrated into the flow of the presentation and case discussion. Patient and provider experience can be enhanced through investing time at the bedside.

Data from the United States show that persons from low socioeconomic backgrounds and those who are socially isolated, belong to racial or ethnic minority groups, or identify as lesbian, gay, bisexual, or transgender experience health disparities at a higher rate. Clinicians must transition from a biomedical to a biopsychosocial framework within the clinical examination to better address social determinants of health that contribute to health disparities. The authors review the characteristics of successful patient-clinician interactions. They describe strategies for relationship-centered care within routine encounters. Our goal is to train clinicians to mitigate differences and reduce disparities in health care delivery.

Telemedicine and telehealth are the practices of medicine at a distance. Performing the equivalent of a complete clinical examination by telemedicine would be unusual. However, components of a more traditional clinical examination are part of the telemedicine workup for specific conditions. Telemedicine clinical examinations are facilitated, and enhanced, through the integration of a class of medical devices referred to as telemedicine peripherals (eg, electronic stethoscopes, tele-ophthalmoscopes, video-otoscopes). Direct-to-consumer telehealth is a rapidly expanding segment of the health care service industry.

Clinical skills remain fundamental to the practice of medicine and form a core component of the professional identity of the physician. However, evidence exists to suggest that the practice of some clinical skills is declining, particularly in the United States. A decline in practice of any skill can lead to a decline in its teaching and assessment, with further decline in practice as a result. Consequently, assessment drives not only learning of clinical skills but also their practice. This article summarizes contemporary approaches to clinical skills assessment that, if more widely adopted, could support the maintenance and reinvigoration of bedside clinical skills.

Physicians can improve their diagnostic acumen by adopting a simulation-based approach to analyzing published cases. The tight coupling of clinical problems and their solutions affords physicians the opportunity to efficiently upgrade their illness scripts (structured knowledge of a specific disease) and schemas (structured frameworks for common problems). The more the number of times clinicians practice accessing and applying those knowledge structures through published cases, the greater the odds that they will have an enhanced approach to similar patient cases in the future. This article highlights digital resources that increase the number of cases a clinician experiences and learns from.

Foreword

Recapturing the Lost Art

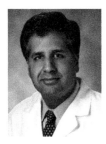

Bimal H. Ashar, MD, MBA, FACP
Consulting Editor

During medical school and residency, I, like many of those likely reading this, was fascinated by physical diagnosis. For me, combining a thorough medical history with an examination that relied upon keen use of the senses to make a diagnosis is what it meant to be a physician. I was in awe of my supervising residents and attendings who pointed out findings that I may have missed. I can remember trying to inspect for signs like Roth spots, splinter hemorrhages, Osler nodes, and Janeway lesions in a patient with suspected infective endocarditis. I went through a phase of searching for ear lobe creases to assess patients' risk for coronary disease and trying to auscultate for posttussive rales in patients with suspected tuberculosis. I distinctly remember the first time I palpated a prostate nodule (admittedly that may be a bit odd).

As time and medicine have *progressed*, the physical examination has become more obsolete. Bedside rounds gave way to "card flipping," which has evolved into rounds with portable laptops outside of patient rooms. In the outpatient setting, patients rarely don gowns in order to maintain efficiency. Practicing physicians likely spend much more time learning how to template out a "comprehensive physical exam" to be able to bill a CPT code 99215 than they do actually reviewing how to perform one. Similarly, time spent palpating and percussing a mouse and keyboard greatly surpasses time with the patient.

It is an honor to have many of the founders and members of the Society of Bedside Medicine collaborate for this issue of the *Medical Clinics of North America*. Dr Garibaldi and his colleagues shed light on the forces surrounding the erosion of

Med Clin N Am 102 (2018) xv–xvi
https://doi.org/10.1016/j.mcna.2018.02.002
0025-7125/18/© 2018 Published by Elsevier Inc.

our clinical skills. More importantly, they provide tools to enhance our diagnostic acumen in our current medical environment.

Bimal H. Ashar, MD, MBA, FACP
Division of General Internal Medicine
Johns Hopkins University School of Medicine
601 North Caroline Street
#7143
Baltimore, MD 21287, USA

E-mail address:
Bashar1@jhmi.edu

Preface

The Clinical Examination in Twenty-First Century Medicine

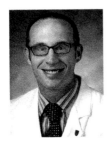

Brian T. Garibaldi, MD
Editor

Clinical medicine has dramatically changed in the century since Sir William Osler established the modern residency system at The Johns Hopkins Hospital in 1889. Our ability to diagnose disease has never been greater. We can predict, and in many cases, prevent illness on an individual and even a population level. Treatment options are expanding and can be specifically tailored to meet an individual patient's needs.

Advances in technology are at the forefront of these exciting developments, but the clinical encounter between a patient and physician remains the cornerstone of medical practice. This time-honored ritual provides the basis for trust and healing for the patient. It is fundamental to accurate diagnosis and high-quality patient-centered care. It is also an important source of fulfillment and satisfaction for the physician. However, a number of factors have challenged the primacy of the clinical encounter in recent years.

Physicians spend less time with patients in the modern hospital and clinic setting. Greater access to technology has shifted the diagnostic process away from the patient and toward the laboratory and radiology suite. While the electronic health record has vast potential, an unintended consequence of its widespread adoption is that providers spend more time caring for the digital representation of a patient (the "i-Patient" as coined by Abraham Verghese and others) than the actual person. Operational constraints on health care such as a focus on throughput and relative value units have also shifted the focus of care away from the bedside.

As a result of these pressures, fundamental clinical skills such as the physical exam are in decline. This erosion in clinical skills is a serious problem. The failure to perform an adequate history and physical exam contributes to unnecessary testing and accounts for a large proportion of diagnostic error. In addition, a decline in clinical skills threatens to erode the physician-patient relationship and likely contributes to the alarming rise in physician burnout. As physical exam skills have declined, so too have the number of practitioners who are confident enough to teach the physical

Med Clin N Am 102 (2018) xvii–xviii
https://doi.org/10.1016/j.mcna.2018.02.001
0025-7125/18/© 2018 Published by Elsevier Inc.

exam. This has led to a spiral in which clinical teaching has increasingly shifted from the bedside into the hallway and conference room, further weakening bedside skills.

In this issue, we explore the enduring value of the clinical encounter, with a particular emphasis on the physical examination. Many of the authors are founders and members of the Society of Bedside Medicine (https://bedsidemedicine.org), an organization dedicated to education, innovation, and research on the role of the clinical encounter in modern medicine. We hope that this issue will inspire all of us to get back to the bedside and provide the tools needed to succeed in both teaching and patient care once we get there.

Brian T. Garibaldi, MD
Co-President, Society of Bedside Medicine
Division of Pulmonary and Critical Care Medicine
Johns Hopkins University School of Medicine
1830 East Monument Street, 5th Floor
Baltimore, MD 21287, USA

E-mail addresses:
bgariba1@jhmi.edu; info@bedsidemedicine.org

The Enduring Value of the Physical Examination

Junaid A.B. Zaman, MA, BMBCh, MRCP[a,b,c,*]

KEYWORDS

- Clinical examination • Bedside medicine • History and physical examination • Value

KEY POINTS

- Physical examination has been a vital tool in medical diagnosis over the last few centuries, but has come under increasing scrutiny because technological aids to diagnosis are thought more reliable.
- It has value beyond diagnostic accuracy, especially in fundamental areas, such as patient safety and cost, and has been shown to improve physician and patient satisfaction with clinical encounters.
- There are certain diagnoses that can only be made by physical examination, and others whereby risk stratification and prognosis are based on physical examination of physiologic function.
- Physical examination complements the increasing technological tools available for bedside diagnosis, and an "either-or" mentality is best avoided.

INTRODUCTION

Physical examination (PE) is defined as "an examination of the bodily functions and condition of an individual."[1] This article focuses exclusively on PE in the context of clinical medicine, that is, the interaction between a health care provider and patient. In short, the title of the article is a statement ratified throughout the article, namely that there is not only benefit (*value*) to PE, but also that it will continue to last (*endure*) for some time. Both "enduring" and "value" are explored in more depth with respect to the future integration of PE into the clinical assessment of a patient and how its value extends well beyond current diagnostic/cost-based metrics.

Disclosure Statement: Funding sources are British Heart Foundation and UK-US Fulbright Commission.
[a] Program for Bedside Medicine, Stanford Hospital, Palo Alto, CA 94305, USA; [b] Department of Cardiology, Good Samaritan Hospital, 616 Witmer Street, Los Angeles, CA 90017, USA; [c] Imperial Centre for Cardiac Engineering, Hammersmith Campus, Du Cane Road, London, W12 0NN, UK
* Program for Bedside Medicine, Stanford Hospital, Palo Alto, CA 94305.
E-mail address: jzaman@stanford.edu

https://doi.org/10.1016/j.mcna.2017.12.003
medical.theclinics.com

EVOLUTION OF THE PHYSICAL EXAMINATION

PE was not always a part of medicine. Its introduction into Western medicine can be traced throughout the last few centuries when novel techniques were applied to aid diagnosis of the sick. It is beyond the remit of this article to detail these discoveries by pioneers of the field (eg, percussion by Auenbrugger or auscultation by Laennec).[2] These discoveries developed into distinct European models of PE and were later incorporated at the bedside by Sir William Osler into the present ritual of *inspection, palpation, percussion, and auscultation*. With his illustrious career spanning Canada (McGill), United States (Pennsylvania, Hopkins), and United Kingdom (Oxford), perhaps nobody was more central than Osler to the modern practice of bedside PE. His bedside philosophy still permeates through teaching at these institutions and beyond. The evolution of PE is superbly reviewed in Refs.[3,4] for those wishing further detail; the pivotal moments are summarized in **Table 1**.

There have always been those who doubt the central role of PE in bedside diagnosis. However, the modern "age of investigations," whereby imaging and laboratory tests are often deemed to have more accuracy than PE maneuvers, presents unique challenges to the primacy of the PE in its current form.[5] Although traditionally thought to lead to approximately 20% of diagnoses[6] (with history comprising 70% and investigations comprising 10%), the dogma of history, examination, investigation is increasingly eroded by hospital workflows whereby much of the initial workup focuses on investigation results, and much of the "H&P" is duplicated from admission clerking. Furthermore, the annual "general physical" for screening in the healthy population is also under attack. Many think it can be replaced by a review of key results and history risk factors and argue this helps improve allocation of health care resources from the well to those who need care.[7]

The division between PE and bedside investigation is increasingly blurred, because electronic instruments such as handheld ultrasound machines allow instant access to advanced imaging. Although some see this clash as an "either/or," predicting the end of the binaural stethoscope as is currently known,[8] there are others who not only use clinical cases to highlight the unique importance of bedside auscultation[9,10] but also

Table 1		
Key developments in the history of the physical examination		
Date	**Person**	**Development**
ca. 400 BC	Hippocrates	Medicine as a profession; disease natural, not divine
ca. AD 1300		Dissection of human bodies increased
1543	Vesalius	*Fabrica* published; first accurate anatomy text
ca. 1670	Sydenham	Classification of disease
1761	Morgagni	*De Sedibus* published. Pathology begins
1761	Auenbrugger	Percussion discovered
1808	Corvisart	Popularization of percussion
1816	Laennec	Stethoscope invented, distributed with each copy of his book
1800–1850	Louis	French School establishes systematic approach to clinical case, still in use to this day
1830–1900	Mueller	German School adds insight from mechanisms of disease, studied by experimental methods
1889	Osler	Medical clinic opens at the Johns Hopkins Hospital

Adapted from Walker HK. The origins of the history and physical examination. In: Walker HK, Hall WD, Hurst JW, editors. Clinical methods: the history, physical, and laboratory examinations. 3rd edition. Boston: Butterworths; 1990. p. 6; with permission.

integrate the use of handheld echo as a PE technique, such as in the Stanford 25.[11] This set of 25 PE maneuvers, techniques, and tips does not exclude the handheld ultrasound, instead actively integrating it into the learning set of modern PE moving away from the dogma of what previously constituted PE. However, it is not only within the definition presented at the start but also a key way to evolve the PE to assimilate technology, rather than appear increasingly estranged from medical progress, which invariably involves new technology.

Another example of how technology is critical to incorporate into PE is the use of video examination during neurologic assessment, as is now often routine for deciding indications for acute thrombolysis of stroke. The observation of asymmetry in facial muscles during speech is as important as proper technique for eliciting reflexes. Such observations can now be done remotely, albeit they may take longer and be less accurate than bedside evaluation.[12] With more and more telemedicine consultations happening globally, this is likely to continue the evolution of the PE to a form that may be significantly different than Osler's time.

KEY ELEMENTS OF A MODERN PHYSICAL EXAMINATION

Despite the evolution of PE, there are key elements that remain unchanged and are worth explicitly stating at this stage to provide a framework for establishing its value.

The first key attribute is that it is patient centered and individual in nature. The ritual of the physician and patient has been eloquently summarized by Abraham Verghese and colleagues[13] and can itself impart significant therapeutic benefit. It cannot be done on multiple patients at once and hence requires the exclusive attention of the examiner. It is a serial, not a parallel activity.

There is great importance placed on consent and good communication in modern medical school training, to allow the patient to feel comfortable during the examination. This may be foregone in medical assessments, which artificially limit history taking and hence diagnostic information to the PE alone, but there is a continuous 2-way dialogue during everyday PE that helps to build rapport between the patient and physician.

Once consented, observation comes first. This is part of the routine of all PE (*inspection*, palpation, percussion, auscultation; *look*, feel, move) and has been popularized in the fiction of Sir Arthur Conan Doyle, who based his detective character Sherlock Holmes on a Scottish surgeon's acute powers of observation. Looking at a patient's scars or gait can give away a diagnosis before any physical contact, something which the trained medical mind assesses during every PE.

Reassurance of the patient that this will not inflict undue suffering or pain is also part of good modern PE. Sometimes it is necessary to elicit a sign, such as guarding, or rebound tenderness, which is unpleasant, but this should be kept to a minimum and the patient forewarned, unless it compromises diagnostic yield. Modern medicine requires chaperones for protection of both examiner and patient in what is otherwise a very vulnerable encounter, with ritual undressing and physical contact crossing boundaries no other stranger is allowed to do routinely.

Two key elements of PE occupy a large proportion of the accumulated literature on PE. The formulation, or reasoning of the signs elicited and how they interact with the history of a given patient, is part of a term called "clinical acumen," which is best learned by the bedside rather than from books. Conversely, the differential diagnosis of a sign or group of findings can be learned from a book, with the bedside experience required to learn the different techniques and ways to obtain reliable, objective data to aid in achieving a diagnosis.

VALUE OF THE PHYSICAL EXAMINATION

The value of the PE is more than just its diagnostic accuracy, although this is the primary outcome in most circumstances. Proper technique in PE requires training (often in small groups), practice, willing patients, and passion on the part of the learner. Improper technique can cause harm and unnecessary suffering, and sometimes, irrevocable loss of trust in the examiner. It is therefore one of the most important skills learned during training. A curious mind set helps to keep these skills evolving throughout an entire career.

The diagnostic value of the PE can in many cases be compared with other modalities such as imaging or other diagnostic testing. This often leads to synergy between the 2 but it is not a mutually exclusive approach. Books such as *Evidence-based Physical Diagnosis*"[14] and journal series such as the *Rational Clinical Examination*[15] proliferate the message that there is a quantitative method of assessing how PE contributes to diagnosis in many common conditions. However, even in the age of technology, the PE remains the diagnostic gold standard for many diseases.

Clinically, there are situations where PE informs prognosis of a patient, such as the Killip classification in NSTEMI[16] or the functional neurologic deficit in determining stroke severity.[17] These are vital to the triage of patients for specialized and often invasive tests. Furthermore, there are "clinical diagnoses" that can *only* be made using PE; these include many neurologic, rheumatologic, and dermatologic conditions.

On a holistic level, PE provides a welcome respite for many physicians from the electronic medical record.[18] Patient contact has benefits for both physicians and patients.[19] These benefits include improved patient ratings of care[20] and reduced physician discontent.[21] Observational data support the pivotal role of PE in guiding diagnosis, therapy, and management, the *sine qua non* of the patient-doctor relationship.[22,23]

In addition, PE reinforces the physician-student relationship, especially in practices where teaching is a large part of daily medical rounds.[24] Personally, the silence as my stethoscope engages my ears and the gradual tuning into the rhythm of the patient's heartbeat is a refreshingly escapist experience every time.

A new conceptual framework for assessing the value of the PE beyond diagnostic positive predictive values, sensitivity, or specificity was recently proposed.[25] These themes are shown in **Fig. 1** and highlight the benefit of PE across many disciplines and to many stakeholders other than the patient.

Most definitions of clinical value include outcome expressed as a function of cost.[26] The 2 key metrics in the framework above which best capture this are patient safety and cost. Given the variability of clinical outcome measures, data on whether PE can directly benefit clinical outcome are limited. However, a recent series of "systematically collected anecdotes" shows how not performing PE was a major factor in medical error,[27] and by inference, patient safety. The denominator, cost, is even more challenging to quantify as the alternative of using technological aids to diagnosis has clearly fixed costs, yet the cost of PE is primarily derived from use of clinician's time. There are few scenarios or studies where the 2 can be compared directly. Judicious use of PE to guide diagnostic tests, especially those with the potential to cause harm, such as exposure to ionizing radiation, will both improve patient safety and reduce cost by allocating resources based on clinical need, improving value from both sides of the outcome/cost equation.

FUTURE OF THE PHYSICAL EXAMINATION

With the rapid development of technology, it is easy to be negative about the role of PE in the future care of patients.[28] It has clearly already suffered a decrease in priority

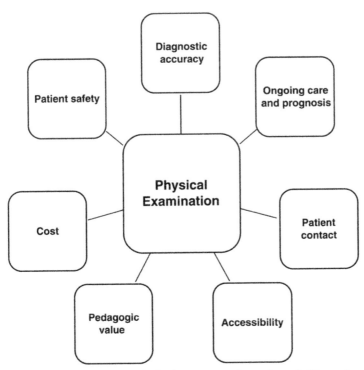

Fig. 1. Seven key parameters by which the comparative value of PE can be assessed. (*Adapted from* Zaman J, Verghese A, Elder A. The value of physical examination: a new conceptual framework. South Med J 2016;109(12):754–7; with permission.)

of medical education, with many residents unable to get away from the "iPatient" on their computer screens and back to the bedside.[29]

This is reflected in current assessments focusing on history (US Medical Licensing Examination [USMLE] step 2 CS) and knowledge base (USMLE steps 1, 2CK). Clinical skills assessment is difficult to standardize, expensive to operationalize, and requires real-life patients. This theme is expertly discussed later in this issue (See "Clinical Skills Assessment in the 21st Century") by Andrew Elder, echoing recent high-profile opinion pieces.[30]

Teaching at the bedside remains the main unit of learning PE. Although it is resource intensive, requiring small groups, it is still highly valued by students and often by patients.[31] The modern development of bite-size teachable moments such as the " 5-minute moment" will help increasingly time-pressured teachers and learners condense learning into a key "nugget" that can be effectively taught in 5 minutes.[32] This special edition of the *Medical Clinics of North America*, conferences such as the Stanford 25 Bedside Clinical Skills Symposium,[33] organizations such as the Society of Bedside Medicine,[34] and a recent report by the Institute of Medicine (now the National Academy of Medicine)[35] confirm this is a high priority for future medical education.

SUMMARY

PE has been integral to development of medicine as it is known. It is likely that some form of patient-physician individual interaction will always be required. PE has utility beyond just cost and diagnostic accuracy. Ideally, it needs assessment to stress importance rather than just "cultural norms." Finally, technology integration should be actively encouraged to keep PE up-to-date with modern medicine.

REFERENCES

1. Anon. Physical examination | definition of physical examination by Merriam-Webster. Merriam Webster. Available at: https://www.merriam-webster.com/dictionary/physical examination. Accessed August 20, 2017.
2. Cummins SL. Auenbrugger and Laennec: the discoverers of percussion and auscultation. Proc R Soc Med 1945;38:409–12. Available at: http://www.ncbi.nlm.nih.gov/pubmed/19993085. Accessed August 20, 2017.
3. Verghese A, Charlton B, Cotter B, et al. A history of physical examination texts and the conception of bedside diagnosis. Trans Am Clin Climatol Assoc 2010; 122:290–311.
4. Walker HK. The origins of the history and physical examination. Boston: Butterworths; 1990. Available at: http://www.ncbi.nlm.nih.gov/pubmed/21250276. Accessed August 20, 2017.
5. Knox R. The fading art of the physical exam. Southern California: NPR; 2010. Available at: http://www.npr.org/templates/story/story.php?storyId=129931999. Accessed August 20, 2017.
6. Campbell EW, Lynn CK. The physical examination. Boston: Butterworths; 1990. Available at: http://www.ncbi.nlm.nih.gov/pubmed/21250202. Accessed August 20, 2017.
7. Mehrotra A, Prochazka A. Improving value in health care — against the annual physical. N Engl J Med 2015;373:1485–7. Available at: http://www.nejm.org/doi/10.1056/NEJMp1507485. Accessed August 20, 2017.
8. Anon. Has the stethoscope had its day? | society | The guardian. Available at: http://www.theguardian.com/society/2016/jan/09/stethoscope-cardiology-doctor-outdated-auscultation. Accessed January 14, 2016.
9. Fuster V. The stethoscope's prognosis: very much alive and very necessary. J Am Coll Cardiol 2016;67(9):1118–9. Available at: http://linkinghub.elsevier.com/retrieve/pii/S0735109716001170.
10. Edelman E, Weber B. Tenuous tether. N Engl J Med 2015;373(23):2199–201.
11. Anon. Stanford medicine 25 | Stanford Medicine 25 | Stanford Medicine. Available at: http://stanfordmedicine25.stanford.edu/. Accessed January 11, 2016.
12. Alasheev AM, Andreev AY, Gonysheva YV, et al. A comparison of remote and bedside assessment of the National Institute of Health Stroke Scale in acute stroke patients. Eur Neurol 2017;77:267–71. Available at: http://www.ncbi.nlm.nih.gov/pubmed/28391278. Accessed September 15, 2017.
13. Verghese A, Brady E, Kapur CC, et al. The bedside evaluation: ritual and reason. Ann Intern Med 2011;155:550–3.
14. McGee S. Evidence-based physical diagnosis. Amsterdam: Elsevier; 2012. Available at: http://www.sciencedirect.com/science/article/pii/B9781437722079000252. Accessed September 7, 2015.
15. Anon. JAMA network | JAMA | the rational clinical examination. Available at: http://jama.jamanetwork.com/collection.aspx?categoryID=6257&page=2. Accessed September 7, 2015.
16. Khot UN, Jia G, Moliterno DJ, et al. Prognostic importance of physical examination for heart failure in non–ST-elevation acute coronary syndromes. JAMA 2003; 290:2174. Available at: http://www.ncbi.nlm.nih.gov/pubmed/14570953. Accessed August 10, 2017.

17. Mukherjee S. A.I. Versus M.D. - The New Yorker. Available at: http://www. newyorker.com/magazine/2017/04/03/ai-versus-md. Accessed August 20, 2017.
18. Kumar AD, Chi J. The illness of present histories. Acad Med 2017;92:1190–1.
19. Chi J, Verghese A. Clinical education and the electronic health record the flipped patient. JAMA 2014;312:2331–2.
20. Kadakia KC, Hui D, Chisholm GB, et al. Cancer patients' perceptions regarding the value of the physical examination: a survey study. Cancer 2014;120:2215–21. Available at: http://www.ncbi.nlm.nih.gov/pubmed/24899511. Accessed September 15, 2017.
21. Mechanic D. Physician discontent. JAMA 2003;290:941. Available at: http://jama. jamanetwork.com/article.aspx?doi=10.1001/jama.290.7.941. Accessed September 15, 2017.
22. Reilly BM. Physical examination in the care of medical inpatients: an observational study. Lancet 2003;362:1100–5. Available at: http://www.sciencedirect. com/science/article/pii/S0140673603144649?via%3Dihub. Accessed September 15, 2017.
23. Kelder JC, Cramer MJ, Van Wijngaarden J, et al. The diagnostic value of physical examination and additional testing in primary care patients with suspected heart failure. Circulation 2011;124:2865–73.
24. Gonzalo JD, Heist BS, Duffy BL, et al. The value of bedside rounds: a multicenter qualitative study. Teach Learn Med 2013;25:326–33. Available at: http://www. ncbi.nlm.nih.gov/pubmed/24112202. Accessed August 20, 2017.
25. Zaman J, Verghese A, Elder A. The value of physical examination: a new conceptual framework. South Med J 2016;109:754–7. Available at: http://sma.org/southern-medical-journal/article/value-physical-examination-new-conceptual-framework. Accessed December 15, 2016.
26. Porter ME. What is value in health care? N Engl J Med 2010;363:2477–81. Available at: http://www.ncbi.nlm.nih.gov/pubmed/21142528. Accessed September 15, 2017.
27. Verghese A, Charlton B, Kassirer JP, et al. Inadequacies of physical examination as a cause of medical errors and adverse events: a collection of vignettes. Am J Med 2015. https://doi.org/10.1016/j.amjmed.2015.06.004.
28. Anon. Dr. Eric topol: digital healthcare will put the patient in charge. Available at: https://www.elsevier.com/connect/Dr-Eric-Topol-Digital-healthcare-will-put-the-patient-in-charge. Accessed August 20, 2017.
29. Verghese A. Culture shock–patient as icon, icon as patient. N Engl J Med 2008; 359:2748–51.
30. Elder A, Chi J, Ozdalga E, et al. The road back to the bedside. JAMA 2013;310: 799–800.
31. Elder AT, Verghese A. Bedside matters - putting the patient at the centre of teaching and learning. J R Coll Physicians Edinb 2015;45:186–7. Available at: http:// www.ncbi.nlm.nih.gov/pubmed/26517094. Accessed January 11, 2016.
32. Chi J, Artandi M, Kugler J, et al. The five minute moment. Am J Med 2016; 129(8):792–5. Available at: http://www.sciencedirect.com/science/article/pii/ S0002934316302091. Accessed March 23, 2016.
33. Anon. Inaugural stanford medicine 25 skills symposium | Department of Medicine | Stanford Medicine. Available at: http://medicine.stanford.edu/2016-report/ inaugural-stanford-medicine-25-skills-symposium.html. Accessed January 11, 2016.
34. Anon. Society of bedside medicine. Available at: https://bedsidemedicine.org/. Accessed September 15, 2017.
35. Balogh EP, Miller BT, Ball JR. Improving diagnosis in health care. Washington, DC: National Academies Press; 2015.

The Physical Examination as Ritual

Social Sciences and Embodiment in the Context of the Physical Examination

Cari Costanzo, PhD[a],*, Abraham Verghese, MD, MACP, FRCP(Edin)[b]

KEYWORDS

- Physical examination • Ritual • Physician-patient relationship • Embodiment
- Social Sciences and Medicine

KEY POINTS

- The privilege of examining a patient is a skill of value beyond its diagnostic utility.
- A thorough physical examination is an important ritual that benefits both patients and physicians; it helps to satisfy a patient's elemental need to be cared for, and a physician's need to make work meaningful.
- The concept of embodiment helps one understand how illness and pain further define and shape the lived experiences of individuals in the context of their race, gender, sexuality, and socioeconomic status.
- A sophisticated understanding of the importance of ritual in medicine, and of placebo effects, reaffirms the significance of the physical examination to the process of building strong physician-patient relationships.

INTRODUCTION

A skilled physical examination in response to a specific patient complaint can be diagnostically effective, allowing one to narrow the differential diagnosis, pluck the "low hanging fruit," and come to a definitive diagnosis. However, in the present era, simple phenotypic observations such as café au lait spots, Horner syndrome, or breast masses are often missed due to a medical culture that does not teach or test bedside skills in the same way that cognitive knowledge is tested and assessed.[1] Furthermore,

Disclosure Statement: Neither author has any relationship with a commercial company that has a direct financial interest in subject matter or materials discussed in article or with a company making a product.
^a Department of Anthropology, Main Quad, Building 50, 450 Serra Mall, Stanford, CA 94305, USA; ^b Department of Medicine, Stanford University, 300 Pasteur Drive S102, Stanford, CA 94305-5110, USA
* Corresponding author.
E-mail address: costanzo@stanford.edu

the physical examination remains underutilized and increasingly threatened by advances in diagnostic testing. As highlighted in the recent Institute of Medicine's report on improving diagnosis in health care, simple oversights in the examination can lead to unnecessary and costly forms of medical error.[2]

The value of the physical examination in building and maintaining the physician-patient relationship is not often studied or discussed. It is telling, however, that patients' complaints about physicians often include words that are revealing of their sense of the importance of the examination and the skill of the person conducting it: "the doctor never touched me!" or "the doctor never laid a hand on me!"[3] The examination of a patient is an honored ritual of caring and healing; the privilege of touch is given to few other professions in society. The authors believe that the failure to connect with patients, the lack of meaningful time spent with patients, and the loss of critical rituals all add to the epidemic of disillusionment and burnout in the medical profession.

A 2016 literature review on the importance of the physical examination points to a disconnect in the medical and social science literature when it comes to the significance and value of the examination in clinical settings.[3] For example, the simple practice of having a patient disrobe can result in feelings that one's identity is being stripped away. The concept of embodiment, as understood through an anthropological lens, can help physicians appreciate anew the importance of the examination and widen its practice. Studies of the neurobiological effects of rituals at the bedside (setting, appearance, tone of voice) suggest that the notion of placebo without a placebo might well apply to the physical examination when it is done with skill and consideration.[1]

Finally, the rapid evolution of artificial intelligence (AI) and deep machine learning will change the landscape even further.[4] AI has great potential to relieve some of what is burdensome in medicine, and it is hoped that if utilized well, and with intelligent input (ie, human intelligence before artificial intelligence, or HI before AI), it may allow for more meaningful patient time. However, certain vital expressions of empathy, understanding, and love remain a unique ritual between human beings, not humans and machines. Human-to-human rituals in medicine benefit not only patients; they also help to relieve the dysphoria and disillusion existing in a medical system that is often technology proficient but emotionally deficient.[5–9]

THE PHYSICAL EXAMINATION IN MEDICINE AND THE SOCIAL SCIENCES

In a 2016 literature review of the physical examination and the physician-patient relationship, Iida and Nishigori identified 1447 studies focused on the physical examination in both the medical and social science databases, selecting 205 studies for further review.[3] They found that although most of the medical literature they reviewed valued the physical examination as a means of building and maintaining the patient-physician relationship, these positive assessments were largely based on opinion rather than quantitative data.[3] Conversely, many existing ethnographic studies of the physical examination highlight the ways that patients often experience such examinations as invasive.[3] These studies unveil power differentials, looking at ways that institutions within society maintain social hierarchies.[10] Simple practices such as using the scientific language of medicine or turning one's back toward a patient to type notes on a computer can feel alienating to a patient, driving a wedge between patients and their physicians. Furthermore, practices like disrobing to don a paper gown can literally strip a patient of his or her identity. What is clearly needed is more scholarship in this area to prospectively assess the importance of the physician-patient relationship. It is the authors' belief that interdisciplinary studies using qualitative and quantitative research methods will shed new light on this subject. The authors also believe that a strong theoretic framework embracing the concept of embodiment will yield a more robust understanding within medicine and the social sciences of the value of the physical examination.

EMBODIMENT

In the 1980s, the concept of embodiment became central to anthropological studies that examined the ways ideologies around sex, gender, and racial differences reinforced systems of oppression in society.[11] The anthropological notion of embodiment rejects the mind/body binary and instead suggests that bodies—and what people think about their bodies—is contingent upon history, culture, and a politics of power. Within this framework, each person's body is situated not only within the story of that individual's life, but also in a larger narrative about how social and political structures have created obstacles or opportunities for different types of bodies in the world. Colonialism, for example, has led to both visible and invisible hierarchies around skin color that have shaped disparate paths for different racial groups in society. The notion of embodiment, therefore, allows one to look holistically at humans in the wider social and political context in which each life is lived. Applied to medicine, the concept of embodiment helps one understand how illness and pain further define and shape the lived experiences of individuals in the context of their race, gender, sexuality, and socioeconomic status.

In a *Companion to the Anthropology of the Body and Embodiment*, Nora Jones encourages readers to think not only about the embodiment of the patient, but also the embodiment of the various stakeholders in medicine. She offers a tripartite framework that looks at (1) the patient's body as seen by the practitioner, (2) the generalized ill or diseased body found in popular culture, and (3) the patient's understanding of his or her own body. Jones refers to this tripartite framework as the body as specimen, spectacle, and patient, respectively.[12]

In an interdisciplinary undergraduate course the authors teach for freshman (many of whom are premedicine), Jones' tripartite framework is used to encourage students to think about what it means to be an embodied human in the modern world. The ability to read the body provides a wider view of the soma than is characteristic of a usual physical diagnosis course. The ability to read the body is, of course, at the center of the physical examination, shaping the way one thinks about individual identities, as well as the future of medicine.[13]

However, even the way a skilled clinician reads the body is never entirely objective; rather it is shaped through the lens of culture at particular moments in history. Culture therefore informs and distorts how one discerns, accepts, rejects, and analyzes one's body. It affects the ways people experience illness, gendered and racialized identities, sexuality, perceptions of beauty, and rights (or lack of rights) to control their own bodies. Some of the fundamental questions that arise when the body is viewed in this fashion are issues of ownership and autonomy (as in the separation of conjoined twins, or a growing surrogacy industry in which poor women in developing nations serve as surrogates for families in developed nations); perceptions of beauty, masculinity and femininity; stigmatization by race and morphology; and limitations that the current gender binary poses for the wider spectrum of lived gender identities, such as transgender or gender fluid.

It is necessary and helpful for medical students and physicians to be reminded of and understand the intersections of identities, and to explore their own cultural biases. For example, in a diverse society, it is not possible to care for, or be a provider who is, a person of color without some deep understanding of how colonialism has led to a hierarchy around skin color in American society, and that hegemony and power often operate in subtle ways to naturalize which types of bodies and identities are entitled to social and political power. The ghost of Tuskegee lingers in the minds of many patients and physicians. Approaching the bedside examination as an important ritual that embraces embodiment within a wider social, cultural, and political history is imperative to building trust between patients and physicians.

THE RITUAL OF THE PHYSICAL EXAMINATION

A ritual typically signifies a rite of passage, the crossing of a threshold, or a sacred event that is marked in contrast to events that are either quotidian or profane. For decades, anthropologists have identified codes of practice that mark rituals as transformative or timeless.[9,14–18] Rituals such as baptism or marriage signify both a sacred event, and a transition in one's social status. So too does the physical examination mark a highly ritualized event. Similarly, a physical examination may also mark a first step toward the crossing of a threshold from sickness to health.[1]

The authors believe the physical examination can be read as a ritual for several reasons:

a. A physical examination typically occurs in a specific, symbolic setting (a doctor's office that contains specialized furniture—namely an examination table—not found in other quotidian or nonmedical spaces).
b. Symbolic tools such as a stethoscope or reflex hammer may be used during a physical examination.
c. The identities and actions of those involved in the ritual remain constant.

One party in the ritual is either a physician, nurse practitioner, or physician assistant, often in a white coat, who lays his or her hands on the patient. The other participant, despite his or her social position (eg, as a homemaker, a software engineer, or a teacher)—dons a neutralizing gown to assume the role of patient. Of course, this potential power imbalance requires extreme diligence on the part of the physician in order to gain and maintain trust with each patient. Disrobing and allowing touch are markers of vulnerability; it is therefore imperative that physicians approach the physical examination attentively and compassionately in order to preserve the embodied identity of their patients.

Furthermore, like all rituals, the ability to pass knowledge from one generation to another—the ability to continue the art and practice of the physical examination—requires hands-on training, or, in effect, an apprenticeship.[1] Efforts such as Stanford 25 training are designed to systematically focus on technique and skill, and impart satisfaction in gaining skill and expanding repertoire.[19] Within medicine, an attending physician guides physicians-in-training at the bedside in order to impart such knowledge. The result of this apprenticeship is twofold; (a) it ensures the survival of the ritual of the physical examination, and (b) it results in the actual patient as the center of attention, rather than focusing on digital images and scans of the patient on a computer, referred to elsewhere as the iPatient.[20] Maintaining the centrality of actual physician-patient interactions is vital to the well-being of patients. Studies in the field of placebo effect are demonstrating that everything that surrounds a pill, such as rituals, symbols, and doctor-patient encounters may in fact have positive neurobiological effects on patients.[21]

THE PLACEBO EFFECT AND THE PHYSICAL EXAMINATION

Studies of placebo—Latin for "I shall please"—have yielded interesting results in pain-drug clinical trials in the last 20 years. In 1996, 27% of patients reported pain reduction from a new drug compared with placebo, but in 2013, that number dropped to only 9%, and not because the drugs were less effective, but because the placebo effect is growing rapidly in the United States.[21] Furthermore, studies of placebo show that it is not just a pill that can have a positive effect; "different social stimuli such as words and rituals of the therapeutic act may change the chemistry and circuitry of a patient's brain."[22] Conversely, there can be a nocebo effect, where negative expectations may in fact make a patient feel worse.[23] Essentially, studies of both placebo and nocebo effects demonstrate that the psychosocial context around patient therapy, such as the ritual around the therapeutic act, can have an effect on the biochemistry of a patient's brain.[23] A well-administered physical examination, for example, can make a patient feel better, while an inferior examination can have a deleterious effect on a patient. Studying the neurobiological effects of the physical examination—treating the physical examination itself as a type of placebo without placebo can help one better understand the importance of the physical examination on the well-being of patients.[24]

Working with 262 randomized patients in a 3-week trial to test the effects of warmth and empathy on patients with irritable bowel syndrome, Kaptchuk and colleagues found that "factors such as warmth, empathy, duration of interaction, and the communication of positive expectation might indeed significantly affect clinical outcome."[25]

Although many studies have shown that social influence affects what people think about a product, Alia Crum in Stanford's Psychology Department conducted a study that tested participant response to uncaffeinated spring water and discovered that social influence can affect people's physiologic reactions to products as well.[26] Crum's research points to the ways that mindset can have an enormous impact on health outcomes.

Crum, Leibowitz, and Verghese argue that placebo effect is "no longer a mysterious response to a sugar pill, but the scaffolding of psychological and social forces—the support system—on which the total effect of treatment rests. Knowing this, we can move beyond merely asking how a treatment compares with a placebo and begin to ask more useful questions such as what are the components driving placebo responses and what can we, as patients and providers, do to more effectively leverage these components to improve healthcare?"[27]

JOY IN PRACTICE AND MEANING IN THE EXAMINATION

Physician burnout is at an all-time high, reaching epidemic proportions as a result of a changing health care system marked by financial pressures, an increased expectation in productivity, the intensified clerical burden required to manage electronic health records (EHR), and new regulatory requirements and levels of scrutiny.[28,29] This has led to a reduction in meaningful time physicians spend with patients. In order to find increased joy in practice, physicians need to feel that the work they are doing is in fact meaningful.[30] In a 2013 study published in the *Annals of Family Medicine*, Sinsky and her colleagues visited 23 high-performing primary-care practices that supported both quality of care and physician work-life balance, looking for factors that brought meaning into their work. Sinsky and her research team found that physician fulfillment "is tightly related to the organization of the practice environment, including relief from paperwork and administrative hassles, the opportunity to form meaningful relationships with patients, and the ability to provide high-quality care to patients."[30] As physicians seek ways to climb out of the massive well of disillusionment and burnout, rituals such as the physical examination—a process that strengthens the physician-patient relationship and adds meaning and joy in practice, will become even more central.

Although advances in AI can automate some processes, perhaps relieving what is burdensome in medicine, it is important that the very aspects of medicine that bring joy and meaning to practice will be retained by human doctors. New AI software might allow machines to recognize certain emotions in human faces, but workers with high emotional skills will remain in high demand.

SUMMARY

The privilege of examining a patient is a skill of value beyond its diagnostic utility. At a time when technology and advances in medicine paradoxically threaten these simple skills, it is important to continue dialogue and research on the value of the focused physical examination. In addition, the aspects of the examination that transcend the usual medical focus—embodiment, identity, power dynamics, symbolism of locating the disease on the body as opposed to on an image or a pathology slide—are as important as ever. At a time when physicians are increasingly disillusioned and experiencing burnout more than ever before, finding meaning is critical, and for most clinicians, it is the interaction with human beings that imparts this meaning. A sophisticated understanding of the importance of ritual in medicine, and of placebo effects, is reaffirming. The authors believe the ritual, when done with skill and consideration, helps satisfy a patient's elemental need to be cared for, and a physician's need to make work meaningful.

REFERENCES

1. Verghese A, Brady E, Kapur CC, et al. Bedside exam: ritual and reason. Ann Intern Med 2011;155(8):550–3.
2. National Academies of Sciences, Engineering, and Medicine. Improving diagnosis in health care. Washington, DC: The National Academies Press; 2015.
3. Iida J, Nishigori H. Physical examination and the physician-patient relationship: a literature review. MedEdPublish; 2016. p. 11–4.
4. Grace K, Salvatier J, Dafoe A, et al. When will AI exceed human performance? Evidence from AI experts. 2017. Available at: https://arxiv.org/pdf/1705.08807. pdf. Accessed May 30, 2017.
5. O'Rourke M. Doctor's tell all—and it's bad. The Atlantic 2014. Available at: https://www.theatlantic.com/magazine/archive/2014/11/doctors-tell-all-and-its-bad/380785/.
6. Jauhar S. Doctored: the disillusionment of an American physician. New York: Farrar, Straus and Giroux; 2014.
7. Lerner BH. The good doctor: a father, a son, and the evolution of medical ethics. Boston: Beacon Press; 2015.
8. Kenney C, Cochran J. The doctor crisis. Philadelphia: Perseus Books Group; 2014.
9. Gawande A. Being mortal. New York: Henry Holt and Company; 2014.
10. Foucault M. Truth and Power. In: Rabinow P, editor. The foucault reader. New York: Pantheon Books; 1984. p. 51–75.
11. Csordas T, editor. Embodiment and experience: the existential ground of culture and self. Cambridge (United Kingdom): Cambridge Univ. Press; 1994.
12. Jones N. BIOETHICS: embodied ethics: from the body as specimen and spectacle to the body as patient. In: Mascia-Lees FE, editor. A companion to the anthropology

of the body and embodiment. Blackwell Publishing; 2011. Available at: http://www.blackwellreference.com/subscriber/tocnode.html?   id=g9781405189491_chunk_g 97814051894917. Accessed March 07, 2017.

13. Jones NL. Embodied Ethics: From the Body as Specimen and Spectacle to the Body as Patient. In: Mascia-Lees FE, editor. A Companion to the Anthropology of the Body and Embodiment. Malden (MA): Wiley-Blackwell; 2011. p. 72–85.

14. Turner V. The ritual process: structure and anti-structure. Ithaca (NY): Cornell University Press; 1969.

15. Bel C. Ritual: perspectives and dimensions. New York: Oxford University Press; 1997.

16. Geertz C. The interpretation of cultures. New York: Basic Books; 1973.

17. Asad T. Toward a genealogy of the concept of ritual, in genealogies of religion. Baltimore (MD): Johns Hopkins University Press; 1993.

18. Douglas M. Purity and danger: an analysis of concepts of pollution and taboo. London: Routledge; 1966.

19. Available at: https://stanfordmedicine25.stanford.edu/.

20. Verghese A. Culture shock—patient as icon, icon as patient. N Engl J Med 2008; 359:2748–51.

21. Resnick B. The weird power of the placebo effect, explained. Vox 2017. Available at: https://www.vox.com/science-and-health/2017/7/7/15792188/placebo-effect-explained.

22. Finniss DG, Kaptchuk TJ, Miller F, et al. Biological, clinical, and ethical advances of placebo effects. Lancet 2010;375:686–95.

23. Frisaldi E, Piedimonte A, Benedetti F. Placebo and nocebo effects: a complex interplay between psychological factors and neurochemical networks. Am J Clin Hypn 2015;57(3):267–84.

24. Benedetti F, Carlino E, Pollo A. How placebos change the patient's brain. Neuropsychopharmacology 2011;36:339–54.

25. Kaptchuck TJ, Kelley JM, Conboy LA, et al. Components of placebo effect: randomised controlled trial in patients with irritable bowel syndrome. BMJ 2008; 336(7651):999–1003. Available at: http://pubmedcentralcanada.ca/pmcc/articles/PMC2364862/pdf/bmj-336-7651-res-00999-el.pdf.

26. Crum AJ, Phillips DJ, Goyer JP, et al. Transforming water: social influence moderates psychological, physiological, and functional response to a placebo product. PLoS One 2016;11(11):e0167121.

27. Crum AJ, Leibowitz KA, Verghese A. Making mindsets matter. BMJ 2017;356: j674.

28. Shanafelt TD, Dyrbye LN, West CP. Addressing physician burnout. The way forward. JAMA 2017;317(9):901–2.

29. Busis NA, Shanafelt TD, Keran CM, et al. Burnout, career satisfaction, and well-being among US neurologists in 2016. Neurology 2017;88(8):797–808.

30. Sinsky C, Willard-Grace R, Schutzbank AM. In search of joy in practice: a report of 23 high functioning primary care practices. Ann Fam Med 2013;11(3):272–8.

The Hypothesis-Driven Physical Examination

Brian T. Garibaldi, MD[a],*, Andrew P.J. Olson, MD[b]

KEYWORDS

- Evidence-based physical diagnosis • Hypothesis-driven physical examination
- Likelihood ratios • Accuracy • Reliability

KEY POINTS

- The physical examination remains a vital part of the clinical encounter.
- Many physical examination maneuvers are just as reliable as diagnostic gold standard tests.
- A hypothesis-driven approach to the physical examination emphasizes the performance of specific physical examination maneuvers that are able to alter the likelihood of disease in a given patient.
- The physical examination should be taught to trainees in a context-specific manner as opposed to the traditional head-to-toe approach.
- Likelihood ratios are diagnostic weights that facilitate interpretation of physical examination findings at the bedside.

INTRODUCTION

For centuries, clinicians have used bedside observation to make diagnostic decisions. Over time, additional modalities have been added to aid in the diagnostic process. Perhaps the greatest example is the introduction of the stethoscope by Laennec in the early nineteenth century.[1] As technology has advanced beyond the stethoscope, diagnosis has moved further away from the bedside in the form of laboratory testing and diagnostic imaging.[2] However, the key to the accurate diagnosis of many conditions still lies in the bedside observations of an astute clinician. In some patients, these observations are the only way to determine the presence or absence of disease (eg, herpes zoster, Parkinson disease, cellulitis, and so forth).[3] In other conditions, additional tests are needed for a definitive diagnosis (eg, myocardial infarction); but the physical examination plays a key role in substantially revising the probability of

Disclosure Statement: The authors have no conflicts of interest to disclose.

[a] Division of Pulmonary and Critical Care, Johns Hopkins University School of Medicine, 1830 East Monument Street, 5th Floor, Baltimore, MD 21205, USA; [b] Division of General Internal Medicine, Department of Medicine, Office of Medical Education, University of Minnesota, 420 Delaware Street Southeast, MMC 284, Minneapolis, MN 55455, USA
* Corresponding author.
E-mail address: bgariba1@jhmi.edu

Med Clin N Am 102 (2018) 433–442
https://doi.org/10.1016/j.mcna.2017.12.005
0025-7125/18/© 2017 Elsevier Inc. All rights reserved.

medical.theclinics.com

disease in order to effectively guide further evaluation. Even after a diagnosis is made, the physical examination is important in following the disease's trajectory and severity. For example, the presence of an S3 gallop in patients with heart failure predicts mortality and might prompt more aggressive intervention beyond the information found on an echocardiogram.[4]

Several Factors Have Led to a Decline in Physical Examination Skills

Despite its enduring importance, several factors have led to a decline in physical examination skills in recent years.[5–7] In the modern hospital, graduate medical trainees spend as little as 12% of their time in direct contact with patients and their families.[8] This lack of time at the bedside has decreased opportunities for deliberate practice and reduced the number of practitioners who are confident in their ability to teach examination skills.[6,9]

There are also many practitioners and learners who question the value and relevance of the physical examination in the age of technology.[10] Some fail to recognize that many physical examination maneuvers are just as reliable as gold standard technology-based tests. Reliability is commonly measured either through simple agreement or by calculating a kappa score. A kappa score of 0 means that agreement between two observers happens by chance alone. A kappa score of 1 indicates perfect agreement. In general, a kappa score greater than 0.4 is considered reasonable for a diagnostic test.[3,11] Many physical examination maneuvers have kappa scores between 0.4 and 0.75, which indicates intermediate to good reliability (**Table 1**). Many diagnostic gold standards have kappa scores that are in that same range. Technology-based tests are not inherently more reliable than the physical examination.

Another reason that some clinicians, particularly those who trained more recently, hold a nihilistic view about the utility of the physical examination is that the examination is often taught as a list of maneuvers to be performed, regardless of the clinical context. Students learn this head-to-toe approach instead of tailoring their examination to each individual patient.[12] They are then assessed on their ability to perform

Table 1
Interobserver reliability (kappa score) for common physical examination findings and common diagnostic standard tests

Physical Finding	Kappa	Diagnostic Standard	Kappa
Liver span >9 cm by percussion	0.11	Classification of coronary artery lesions (by catheterization)	0.33
Delayed carotid upstroke	0.26	Pulmonary infiltrate (by chest radiograph)	0.38
Diminished cardiac dullness	0.49	Cardiomegaly (by chest radiograph)	0.48
Facial palsy (present or absent)	0.57	Severity of valvular regurgitation (by echo)	0.32–0.55
Clubbing (Schamroth sign)	0.64	Cirrhosis (by liver biopsy)	0.59
Systolic hypertension (SBP >160 mm Hg)	0.75	Calf DVT (by ultrasound)	0.69
Tachycardia (pulse >100 bpm)	0.85	Diagnosis of narrow complex tachycardia (by ECG)	0.70
Abdominal jugular test	0.92	Interstitial edema (by chest radiograph)	0.83

Abbreviations: bpm, beats per minute; DVT, deep venous thrombosis; ECG, electrocardiogram; echo, echocardiogram; SBP, systolic blood pressure.

Adapted from McGee S. Reliability of physical findings. In: McGee S, editor. Evidence-based physical diagnosis. 4th edition. Philadelphia: Elsevier; 2018. p. 13; with permission.

the maneuvers on this extensive list. This approach is in stark contrast to how other diagnostic tests are taught and obtained and is an approach that is increasingly frowned on in the age of precision medicine.[13,14] Imagine if medical students were encouraged to obtain a complete blood count, comprehensive metabolic panel, and coagulations studies in every patient in order to be thorough rather than tailoring their diagnostic evaluation. It is not at all surprising, then, that some learners find the physical examination to be less useful than other diagnostic tests.

Clinicians Tailor the Physical Examination to Each Individual Patient in a Hypothesis-Driven Fashion

Although the physical examination is taught and learned in a head-to-toe manner, this is rarely the way in which the examination is actually performed at the bedside. Clinicians in practice perform selected maneuvers in a sequence that is choreographed for each patient. Take, for example, the difference between the clinic room examination for a patient presenting with shortness of breath versus the examination for a patient with knee pain. Clinicians tailor their examination to the individual likelihood of various diseases in each patient and perform maneuvers that are likely to revise these probabilities. This approach to the physical examination is referred to as the hypothesis-driven physical examination (HDPE). Such a framework that encourages the application of the physical examination in a directed, tailored approach instead of a rote, acontextual manner can make the physical examination more useful and decrease unnecessary clinical testing.

We can all think of examples where an unexpected finding on a thorough physical examination has led to a correct and previously unconsidered diagnosis. This approach is particularly valuable in patients who are unable to provide a clear history (eg, patients with altered mental status, critically ill patients in the intensive care unit, and so forth) and in patients with a complex disease or unexplained symptoms in which there is a high level of diagnostic uncertainty and when myriad diagnoses are realistically being considered. In addition to uncovering important and unsuspected findings, performing a thorough physical examination in such patients often helps providers shift from system 1 to system 2 thinking as discussed in Bennett W. Clark and colleagues' article, "Diagnostic Errors and the Bedside Clinical Examination," in this issue. But this complete physical examination is actually a hypothesis-driven process where maneuvers are performed with anticipation for their results, rather than just going through the motions. The HDPE can resemble a complete physical examination under the right circumstances.

There is tremendous value in the physical examination for both patients and providers that goes beyond its ability to diagnose disease. There is an immeasurable sacredness and intimate vulnerability that occurs during a physical examination. As described in Cari Costanzo and Abraham Verghese's article, "The Physical Exam as Ritual: Social Sciences and Embodiment in the Context of the Physical Exam," in this issue, the physical examination is a ritual that in and of itself may have therapeutic properties for both patients and physicians alike. A well-performed physical examination may be beneficial, but a hastily or poorly performed examination has the potential to cause harm.[2,15] A hypothesis-based approach to the physical examination requires that clinicians abandon physical examination maneuvers that have been shown to have little, if any, diagnostic utility and may, in fact, be harmful (eg, the screening pelvic examination in asymptomatic patients).[16] By eliminating maneuvers that lack diagnostic value, the examination will be more useful and efficient, while still preserving the important social and cultural aspects of the physical examination as ritual.

BASICS OF THE HYPOTHESIS-DRIVEN PHYSICAL EXAMINATION

The performance of the HDPE can be separated into 3 tasks that can be then integrated into the whole task of a patient encounter (or simulated encounter for learning). First, accurate pretest probabilities for the likelihood of possible conditions in each patient must be considered. Second, physical examination maneuvers that have adequate operating characteristics to revise the probability of disease should be selected and performed. Lastly, the results of these findings must be combined with the respective pretest probability in order to arrive at a posttest probability. This will allow the creation of a prioritized differential diagnosis to guide the remainder of the evaluation. The authors discuss this process in more detail later.

Determination of Pretest Probabilities

One of the foundational aspects to making accurate, timely diagnoses is the determination of pretest probabilities for specific conditions; these are the probabilities that are revised during history taking and the physical examination. Overestimation or underestimation of pretest probability during diagnostic evaluation may lead to expenditure of cognitive and clinical resources on improbable diagnostic hypotheses. This issue is called base-rate neglect and is one of the most important factors in diagnostic error.[17] Pretest probability can be determined using published data on the epidemiology of a disease, but it can also be modified based on a clinician's personal experience with a given population or in a certain practice. For example, a 65-year-old man with a 3-month history of progressive cough who is referred to an interstitial lung disease clinic at a tertiary care center is much more likely to have idiopathic pulmonary fibrosis than postnasal drip. This prevalence estimate is critical when evaluating the significance of test results. The pretest probability of some diagnostic considerations are orders of magnitude higher than others and should be given more initial diagnostic consideration.

Using Likelihood Ratios to Select Appropriate Physical Examination Maneuvers

In order for the HDPE to be maximally effective, clinicians must focus on performing maneuvers that have the best operating characteristics to revise the probability of a particular diagnostic hypothesis. Cognitive load is limited by this narrowing of focus, and more attention may be paid to the test's findings rather than its performance alone.[18,19]

How can we best understand which physical examination maneuvers have the most discriminatory/diagnostic value? In addition to understanding the reliability of a test (ie, its reproducibility from one examiner to another), a compelling, and pragmatic, answer lies in the concept of likelihood ratios (LRs).[20] Some physical examination findings when present change the likelihood that patients have a disease. These findings are called positive LRs (LR+). For example, the finding of delayed carotid pulses increases the likelihood of aortic stenosis in patients with a systolic ejection murmur. Other physical examination findings when absent change the likelihood that patients have a disease. These factors are called negative LRs (LR−). This terminology can be confusing because both LR+ and LR− can increase or decrease the probability of disease. For example, the *presence* of an early peaking murmur *decreases* the likelihood of severe aortic stenosis in patients with a systolic ejection murmur. Similarly, the *absence* of radiation to the neck, *decreases* the likelihood of aortic stenosis.[3]

LRs are derived from the sensitivity and specificity of the examination maneuver. The sensitivity of a physical examination maneuver refers to the proportion of patients who have the disease who have the physical finding. Specificity refers to the proportion of patients without the disease who lack the physical examination finding. In general, a highly sensitive test when absent, decreases the likelihood of a disease. A highly specific test when present, increases the likelihood of disease. When visually displayed, one can see why sensitivity and specificity are used for decreasing and increasing likelihood, respectively (**Fig. 1**). A more sensitive test has fewer false negatives (and, thus, a negative test is likely to be a true negative), whereas a more specific test has fewer false positives (and, thus, a positive test is likely to be a true positive).

LRs combine these two performance characteristics. A positive LR is the number of patients with the disease who have the finding divided by the number of patients without the disease who have the finding (ie, the sensitivity divided by [1 − specificity]). A negative LR is the number of patients with the disease who do not have the finding, divided by the number of patients without with disease who do not have the finding (ie, [1 − sensitivity] divided by specificity). For an excellent explanation of LRs, please refer to Stephen McGee's text, *Evidence-Based Physical Diagnosis*.[3]

A

	Disease Present	Disease Absent
Test Positive	60	10
Test Negative	40	90
	Sensitivity 60%	Specificity 90%

B

	Disease Present	Disease Absent
Test Positive	90	40
Test Negative	10	60
	Sensitivity 90%	Specificity 60%

Fig. 1. Changes in sensitivity and specificity change false-positive and false-negative rates. (*A*) In tests with higher specificity, the false-positive rate is lower (compare *light gray boxes* in [*A*] and [*B*]). A positive test makes the diagnosis more likely. (*B*) In tests with higher sensitivity, the false-negative rate is lower (compare *dark gray boxes* in [*A*] and [*B*]). A negative test makes the diagnosis less likely.

Arriving at a Posttest Probability

If you have already estimated the pretest probability of a disease, you can apply a specific examination maneuver and, based on the presence of absence of a finding, you can determine the posttest probability of disease. LRs greater than 1 increase the posttest probability, whereas LRs less than 1 decrease the posttest probability. Calculating actual posttest probability is beyond the scope of this article, but there are a few helpful tips that allow the use of LRs at the bedside without complex calculations. A LR of 1 does not change the pretest probability, so a physical examination finding with an LR of 1 does not help in making a diagnosis. For example, Homans sign for detecting calf vein deep venous thrombosis has an LR of approximately 1 and is not helpful in ruling in or ruling out that diagnosis.[21] LRs of 2, 5, and 10 increase the pretest probability by 15%, 30%, and 45%, respectively. LRs of 0.5, 0.2, and 0.1 decrease the pretest probability by 15%, 30%, and 45%, respectively. Physical examination LRs are essentially diagnostic weights that either increase or decrease the probability of disease (**Fig. 2**).[3,20]

There are several useful resources that provide the prevalence of common diseases as well as the LRs for common physical examination findings.[3,22]

Using Hypothesis-Driven Physical Examination in Practice

The use of HDPE in clinical practice is best illustrated by a case. Imagine that you are seeing a 64-year-old former smoker for a routine health visit. He asks you if he might have chronic obstructive pulmonary disease (COPD). The prevalence of COPD in adults in the United States who ever smoked is estimated to be 22%.[23] On chest examination, he has absence of superficial cardiac dullness at the left lower sternal border. The LR for the finding of absent cardiac dullness at the left lower sternal border indicating COPD is approximately 10.[3] The posttest probability of COPD in this patient based on that finding would be 67% (pretest probability of 22% + 45% [the increase in probability associated with a LR of 10]). This posttest probability is high enough to warrant further diagnostic evaluation and may be an effective piece of information to positively inform smoking cessation counseling and to select disease-specific therapies.

The finding of absent cardiac dullness on anterior chest percussion is an underutilized physical examination maneuver. In addition to having a high LR, it is also a test with moderate reliability (kappa = 0.49).[24] Many clinicians do not routinely perform anterior chest percussion. However, in the appropriate context it can provide significant diagnostic value. In contrast, percussing diaphragmatic excursion is a maneuver that is commonly taught to medical students that provides no significant diagnostic value when trying to determine if patients have COPD. In the case of suspected COPD, percussion of diaphragmatic excursion could be confidently omitted, much to the chagrin of the clinical skills course preceptor.

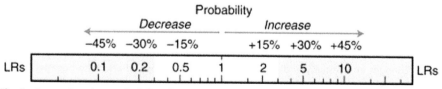

LRs = Diagnostic Weights

Fig. 2. Approximating probability. (*From* McGee S. Diagnostic accuracy of physical findings. In: McGee S, editor. Evidence-based physical diagnosis. 4th edition. Philadelphia: Elsevier; 2018. p. 13; with permission.)

IMPORTANT CAVEATS FOR THE USE OF LIKELIHOOD RATIOS
Not All Examination Maneuvers Have Associated Likelihood Ratios

It is important to note that not all examination maneuvers have reported LRs. For example, if the presence of a physical examination finding defines the disease (ie, it is the gold standard test), there will not be an associated LR. Think of a patient with a herpes zoster rash. One does not need to calculate pretest or posttest probabilities of disease if the rash is characteristic; the patient has zoster. There are also examination maneuvers for which robust LR data are not available. This lack of data does not mean that the examination maneuver has no value and should not be performed; that maneuver needs to be interpreted in the context of the individual patient and the findings considered based on experience and the best available evidence.

Using Multiple Examination Findings to Calculate Posttest Probability

Clinicians usually perform several different physical examination maneuvers when considering a diagnosis. When multiple examination maneuvers are performed, the LRs of each individual maneuver can probably be added together, as long as it is reasonable to assume that the findings are physiologically independent. This is oftentimes not the case, and this approach will likely overestimate the posttest probability of disease. Consider a 77-year-old patient who is referred to you because of a cardiac murmur that was heard during a recent hospitalization for urosepsis. You are concerned about possible aortic stenosis. On physical examination, you hear a mid to late peaking systolic ejection murmur that radiates to the carotids and note that he has delayed carotid upstrokes. The findings of delayed carotid upstrokes and a late peaking murmur each have LRs favoring the diagnosis of aortic stenosis.[3] However, both findings are caused by obstruction to blood flow at the level of a stenotic aortic valve. It would not be fair to add their LRs together to determine the final posttest probability of disease because the findings have the same pathophysiologic basis. It would probably be more appropriate to take the larger of the two LRs and use that to calculate posttest probability.

In contrast, when examination findings are physiologically independent, they can likely be combined to modify posttest probability. For example, jaundice and splenomegaly are physiologically independent (the former arising from hepatic synthetic dysfunction and the latter arising from portal hypertension). These findings could be reasonably combined to revise the probability that a patient has cirrhosis.

One way to confidently use multiple examination maneuvers is to look for studies that have identified independent findings and combined them into prediction rules or "stop rules."[20] A recent and highly successful version of a stop rule is the HINTS (head-impulse test, direction-changing nystagmus, and test of skew) test for patients who present with acute dizziness. If a patient with acute dizziness has an abnormal head impulse test (implying a peripheral cause of vertigo), and no direction-changing nystagmus or skew deviation (both findings that imply a central cause of vertigo), the LR for an acute stroke is 0.02. This LR is better than the LR of a normal diffusion-weighted MRI in ruling out acute stroke.[3,25] Other well-known examples are the Wells score for venous thromboembolism[26] and the Centor criteria for streptococcal pharyngitis.[27] Clinical prediction rules have the advantage of being more predictive than the individual tests they contain.

TEACHING THE HYPOTHESIS-DRIVEN PHYSICAL EXAMINATION
The Concept of Coselection

In addition to routinely performing more than one examination maneuver during a patient encounter, clinicians usually consider more than one diagnosis at a time. The process by which multiple potential diagnoses are considered and evaluated is called coselection. Instead of creating diagnostic hypotheses after the history and physical examination (as is done in many morning reports), the HDPE encourages clinicians to consider diagnostic hypotheses before and during the application of history and physical examination maneuvers. This practice makes intuitive sense. Information obtained from the history guides additional questions and relevant physical examination maneuvers. The information obtained on the physical examination prompts new avenues of questioning as well as additional physical examination maneuvers.

Although this is a process that many physicians conduct intuitively, there is concern that the cognitive load of coselection may be too great for trainees, who are learning the maneuvers at the same time they are learning the clinical context. Some of the cognitive load can be decreased by limiting the number of diagnostic hypotheses during simulation and early clinical experiences.[28] This strategy is likely good for practicing clinicians as well: focusing on a few key potential diagnoses is a more doable task than considering many diagnoses without focused attention. Focusing physical examination training on key findings that discriminate between different diagnoses can also reduce the cognitive load for learners.[28]

Medical Education Training Programs and Hypothesis-Driven Physical Examination

Medical education training programs should encourage mastery of physical examination maneuvers with proven or potential diagnostic utility and should de-emphasize maneuvers that lack diagnostic value. Examples of tests that should not be taught or routinely performed include Homans sign for diagnosing deep vein thrombosis[3,21] and Tinel's sign for diagnosing carpel tunnel syndrome.[29] These tests lack discriminative value and are not helpful in changing the likelihood of disease. In addition, when another diagnostic modality (such as point-of-care ultrasound) is clearly superior to an existing physical diagnosis maneuver for the question at hand, clinicians should adapt their practice, when possible, to include that additional testing modality. Training programs at the undergraduate and graduate level should also incorporate newer diagnostic modalities. The physical examination is not in competition with technology; in many cases, they provide the most valuable information when used together.

A reflective approach that emphasizes discriminatory features improves learners' diagnostic performance in simulated cases. This approach asks learners to identify what features for a given diagnostic hypothesis are present and expected, which features are expected but absent, and which features are present and unexpected. Early research shows that the concerns about students' inability to learn and perform the physical examination in a hypothesis-driven manner are likely unfounded. First-year medical students naturally perform the physical examination in a hypothesis-driven, patient-tailored manner when allowed to do so during a clinical skills examination.[12] This finding is striking given that first-year students have little, if any, contextual clinical knowledge.

SUMMARY

The physical examination remains a vital part of the clinical encounter. For some diagnoses, the physical examination remains the gold standard diagnostic test. For other diagnoses, the physical examination provides prognostic information above and beyond technologically based tests. Although some physicians think that technology is more reliable than bedside observation, this is simply not true for several important physical examination maneuvers. When faced with a clinical question, it is most often not practical to perform every head-to-toe physical examination maneuver from medical school in the hopes of finding something relevant. Physicians select particular aspects of the examination that will likely be important to the issue at hand. This approach is often done intuitively based on experience and prior training. However, a more intentional focus on examination maneuvers that are accurate and reliable can greatly increase the efficiency and diagnostic yield of the physical examination. The HDPE is a valuable tool to practice and teach a high-yield approach to bedside clinical examination and is part of a growing movement to return practitioners and trainees to the bedside.[6,7,30]

REFERENCES

1. Tomos I, Karakatsani A, Manali ED, et al. Celebrating two centuries since the invention of the stethoscope: RenéThéophile hyacinthe laënnec (1781-1826). Ann Am Thorac Soc 2016;13(10):1667–70.
2. Zaman J, Verghese A, Elder A. The value of physical examination: a new conceptual framework. South Med J 2016;109(12):754–7.
3. McGee S. Evidence-based physical diagnosis. Philadelphia: Elsevier; 2018.
4. Likoff MJ, Chandler SL, Kay HR. Clinical determinants of mortality in chronic congestive heart failure secondary to idiopathic dilated or to ischemic cardiomyopathy. Am J Cardiol 1987;59(6):634–8.
5. Vukanovic-Criley JM, Hovanesyan A, Criley SR, et al. Confidential testing of cardiac examination competency in cardiology and noncardiology faculty and trainees: a multicenter study. Clin Cardiol 2010;33(12):738–45.
6. Garibaldi BT, Niessen T, Gelber AC, et al. A novel bedside cardiopulmonary physical diagnosis curriculum for internal medicine postgraduate training. BMC Med Educ 2017;17(1):182.
7. Elder A, Verghese A. Bedside medicine: back to the future? South Med J 2016; 109(12):736–7.
8. Block L, Habicht R, Wu A, et al. In the wake of the 2003 and 2011 duty hours regulations, how do internal medicine interns spend their time? J Gen Intern Med 2013;28(8):1042–7.
9. Russell SW, Garibaldi BT. The other sylvian fissure: exploring the divide between traditional and modern bedside rounds. South Med J 2016;109(12):747–9.
10. Bergl P, Farnan JM, Chan E. Moving toward cost-effectiveness in physical examination. Am J Med 2015;128(2):109–10.
11. Gordis L. Assessing the validity and reliability of diagnostic and screening tests. In: Epidemiology. 5th edition. Philadelphia: Elsevier Saunders; 2014.
12. Allen S, Olson A, Menk J, et al. Hypothesis-driven physical examination curriculum. Clin Teach 2016;14(6):417–22.
13. Mirnezami R, Nicholson J, Darzi A. Preparing for precision medicine. N Engl J Med 2012;366(6):489–91.
14. Collins FS, Varmus H. A new initiative on precision medicine. N Engl J Med 2015; 372(9):793–5.
15. Verghese A, Brady E, Kapur CC, et al. The bedside evaluation: ritual and reason. Ann Intern Med 2011;155(8):550–3.
16. Bloomfield HE, Olson A, Greer N, et al. Screening pelvic examinations in asymptomatic, average-risk adult women: an evidence report for a clinical practice guideline from the American College of Physicians. Ann Intern Med 2014; 161(1):46–53.
17. Croskerry PMDP. The importance of cognitive errors in diagnosis and strategies to minimize them. Acad Med 2003;78(8):775–80.

18. Van Merriënboer JJG, Sweller J. Cognitive load theory in health professional education: design principles and strategies. Med Educ 2010;44(1):85–93.
19. Chen R, Grierson L, Norman G. Manipulation of cognitive load variables and impact on auscultation test performance. Adv Health Sci Educ Theory Pract 2015;20(4):935–52.
20. McGee S. Teaching evidence-based physical diagnosis: six bedside lessons. South Med J 2016;109(12):738–42.
21. Vaccaro P, Van Aman M, Miller S, et al. Shortcomings of physical examination and impedance plethysmography in the diagnosis of lower extremity deep venous thrombosis. Angiology 1987;38(3):232–5.
22. Simel DL, Rennie D. The rational clinical examination: evidence-based clinical diagnosis. New York: McGraw-Hill; 2009.
23. Celli BR, Halbert RJ, Nordyke RJ, et al. Airway obstruction in never smokers: results from the Third National Health and Nutrition Examination Survey. Am J Med 2005;118(12):1364–72.
24. Badgett RG, Tanaka DJ, Hunt DK, et al. Can moderate chronic obstructive pulmonary disease be diagnosed by historical and physical findings alone? Am J Med 1993;94(2):188–96.
25. Kattah JC, Talkad AV, Wang DZ, et al. HINTS to diagnose stroke in the acute vestibular syndrome. three-step bedside oculomotor examination more sensitive than early MRI diffusion-weighted imaging. Stroke 2009;40(11):3504–10.
26. Wells PS, Anderson DR, Bormanis J, et al. Value of assessment of pretest probability of deep-vein thrombosis in clinical management. Lancet 1997;350(9094): 1795–8.
27. Centor RM, Witherspoon JM, Dalton HP, et al. The diagnosis of strep throat in adults in the emergency room. Med Decis Making 1981;1(3):239–46.
28. Bordage G. Why did I miss the diagnosis? Some cognitive explanations and educational implications. Acad Med 1999;74(10):S138–43.
29. D'Arcy CA, McGee S. Does this patient have carpal tunnel syndrome? JAMA 2000;283(23):3110–7.
30. The Society of Bedside Medicine. 2017. Available at: https://bedsidemedicine. org/. Accessed October 9, 2017.

The Role of Technology in the Bedside Encounter

Andre Kumar, MD[a], Gigi Liu, MD, MSc[b], Jeff Chi, MD[a], John Kugler, MD[a],*

KEYWORDS

• Technology • Point-of-care ultrasound • Bedside medicine • Physical examination

KEY POINTS

• Technology has the ability to both strengthen and weaken the patient-physician relationship.
• The electronic health record has become a source of distraction from the bedside encounter, but it does not need to be.
• Point-of-care ultrasound is the most exciting way to bring physicians back to the bedside.
• Future technology needs to be implemented in ways that strengthen the patient-physician relationship.

Technology impacts nearly every aspect of modern life. Much of the technology that is used in our modern health care system is remote from patients and the patient care experience. It is the technology used in making new pharmaceuticals, new medical devices, new laboratory tests, and improved medical imaging. This technology is mostly hidden from patients as they receive care but makes headlines as society grapples with the cost of developing and implementing this new technology, such as with the combination drug ledipasvir/sofosbuvir for hepatitis C treatment.[1] This article looks to examine how technology is affecting the clinical encounter in both positive and negative ways for patients and physicians. The authors hope to show that technology, specifically point-of-care ultrasound, can be used to enhance the patient-physician relationship and the care provided at the patients' bedside.

Initial technologic developments, such as the stethoscope, brought physicians and patients closer together. Diagnoses were made in real time during the patient encounter. This practice changed as medicine moved into the modern era and new technology, especially laboratory and imaging technology, was used remotely from the bedside. Patients today need to wait for laboratory and pathology results or imaging reads to receive a diagnosis and a plan of care. Results are relayed over the phone, via electronic patient portals, during future visits, or sometimes not at all.[2] The development of

Disclosure Statement: No authors have any financial relationships to disclose.
[a] Department of Medicine, Division of Hospital Medicine, Stanford University, mail code 5209, 300 Pasteur Drive, Stanford, CA 94305, USA; [b] Department of Medicine, Johns Hopkins University, 600 North Wolfe Street, Meyer Building 8th Floor, Room 147, Baltimore, MD 21204, USA
* Corresponding author.
E-mail address: jkugler@stanford.edu

Med Clin N Am 102 (2018) 443–451
https://doi.org/10.1016/j.mcna.2017.12.006
0025-7125/18/© 2018 Elsevier Inc. All rights reserved.

point-of-care ultrasound is reversing this trend, allowing the treating physician to expand the physical examination and improve bedside decision-making in real time. In the article "Tenuous Tether" the investigators speak of the importance of the stethoscope in binding physicians to patients: "Devices that bring us closer to the bed breathe new life into our roles as healers."[3] Although the investigators spoke of the stethoscope, the authors see how this equally applies to point-of-care ultrasound. In contrast, devices that take us away from patients have the potential to distract physicians from our roles as healers. The electronic health record (EHR) is an example of a potential distraction and is discussed in more detail (See Helene F. Hedian's article, "The Electronic Health Record and the Clinical Examination," in this issue for further details).

With the introduction of the EHR and time-saving functions like templates and copy/paste, physicians are suddenly able to document large quantities of notes in a fraction of the time. The ability to access the medical record from any location, even from outside the hospital, has eliminated the need to search for physical charts. Laboratory test results and vitals for multiple patients can also be quickly reviewed within a short period of time. Despite these advances, time-in-motion studies have consistently shown that physicians and trainees spend a significant proportion of their time at the computer interacting with the EHR.[4] Time-intensive EHR tasks include chart review and data review, reflecting the exponential growth of documentation and laboratory data that have become prevalent in today's health care landscape.[5] Accordingly, trainees are becoming accustomed to prioritizing EHR data ahead of information gathered directly from patients,[6] in contrast to the more traditional workflow of meeting patients first. This behavior has caused senior physicians to lament the evolving practice of medicine in the modern era, noting that physicians today spend more time in front of the screen, as opposed to time with patients.[7] Although the EHR has often been cited as a detractor of direct patient contact at the bedside, it is interesting to note that time-in-motion studies predating the advent of the EHR also showed that physicians spent a significant amount of time engaged in indirect care.[8] Perhaps the increasing use of computers in the health care workspace has suddenly made physicians more aware of the amount of indirect care for which they are responsible.

When used with a patient focus, rather than allowing the EHR to separate physicians and patients, it can be incorporated at the bedside in a way that facilitates communication.[9] Mobile platforms and portable computers can be used to share imaging and patient data in ways that include patients in medical decision-making and promote awareness and engagement. In this way the EHR, which is often vilified for distracting from patients, could become a way to strengthen the relationship between the physician and patients.

Point-of-care ultrasound has the potential to reverse the trend of technology pulling physicians away from the bedside. Point-of-care ultrasound can be defined as limited ultrasound examinations performed by the treating clinician to make real-time decisions. It is different from traditional radiology- or cardiology-performed studies because the images are not obtained by a technician (ie, sonographer or echocardiographer) and interpreted later by a physician, but rather it is performed and interpreted by the treating clinician.[10] The studies are generally termed *limited* because they tend to be less ambitious than traditional radiology and cardiology studies. Ideally, point-of-care ultrasound studies should be used to answer limited and specific diagnostic questions. This reflects the fact that most point-of-care ultrasound users have significantly less training and expertise than the specialists who read ultrasound images as well as the fact that point-of-care ultrasound machines tend to have lower resolution when compared with traditional ultrasound machines. For example, a point-of-care ultrasound study may be used to evaluate for the presence of a pericardial effusion but would be a poor choice to look for the vegetations of endocarditis.

FOCUSED ASSESSMENT WITH SONOGRAPHY IN TRAUMA

Emergency medicine has been a pioneer and driver of point-of-care ultrasound technology. In a field where decisions frequently need to be made quickly, point-of-care ultrasound is a natural fit. The focused assessment with sonography in trauma (FAST) examination was an early study that gained wide adoption within the emergency medicine community. The FAST examination is used to assess for intra-abdominal injury after blunt or penetrating abdominal trauma. FAST uses ultrasound primarily to find free fluid in the abdomen and has largely replaced diagnostic peritoneal lavage to assess for hemoperitoneum. The FAST examination is done as part of the trauma assessment, performed by both emergency medicine and trauma surgery physicians. Depending on the study, the test characteristics vary with generally high sensitivity but less specificity.[11–14] A systematic review of articles about intra-abdominal injury and ultrasound noted that the FAST examination is a sensitive and specific test that can be performed to assess for intra-abdominal injury using computed tomography (CT) of the abdomen as the gold standard. In this review, a positive FAST examination had a likelihood ratio (LR) of 82 if studies included hemodynamically unstable patients and an LR of 36 if the studies excluded hemodynamically unstable patients. A negative FAST examination in studies that included hemodynamically unstable patients had a negative LR of 0.16. If hemodynamically unstable patients were excluded, the negative LR was 0.33.[15] This review points out that a negative FAST examination in stable patients decreases the likelihood of intra-abdominal bleeding or injury, whereas a positive study essentially confirms the diagnosis. As with every examination the authors review, clinical judgment and incorporation of all the available clinical evidence is essential and best performed by the clinician at the bedside.

The FAST examination is rarely used by internal medicine because it is a trauma-specific study. Internal medicine first began to use point-of-care ultrasound for procedural guidance.

POINT-OF-CARE ULTRASOUND FOR PROCEDURAL GUIDANCE

Point-of-care ultrasound for procedural guidance is now considered the standard of care for central venous access,[16,17] thoracentesis,[18] and paracentesis.[19] The use of ultrasound to guide peripheral venous cannulation increases success rate and reduces the number of central venous catheters.[20,21] A comprehensive review of the use of ultrasound for procedural guidance is beyond the scope of this article.

DIAGNOSTIC POINT-OF-CARE ULTRASOUND

Point-of-care ultrasound was first used by most internal medicine physicians for procedure guidance; however, in more recent years pocket ultrasounds are being used for diagnostic studies and are transforming the way many physicians conduct the physical examination.

CARDIAC

Point-of-care echocardiography is perhaps the most widely used point-of-care ultrasound assessment. It has been adopted by several major society guidelines, including critical care,[22] emergency medicine,[23] and cardiology.[24] Point-of-care echo as opposed to a traditional echo study is more limited in scope, focuses on qualitative rather than quantitative evaluations, and should ideally address a binary question (eg, Is the LV function normal?). Bedside echocardiography focuses on 4 standardized views: parasternal long axis, parasternal short axis, apical 4 chamber, and subcostal.

With minimal training, physicians can reliably identify ventricular function, gross valvular abnormalities, and pericardial effusions and provide accurate assessments of intravascular volume status.[22]

Systolic Function

Point-of-care assessments of right ventricular (RV) and left ventricular (LV) systolic function vary from qualitative assessments using multiple views[24] to formal methodologies that require the measurement of end-systolic and end-diastolic volume in 2 planes.[22] Even among physicians with minimal training, qualitative assessments of reduced LV ejection fraction (LVEF) are reliable, with a reported sensitivity and specificity as high as 94% for identifying patients with a moderately reduced LVEF.[22,25] However, a qualitative assessment of LVEF requires multiple views; several factors (eg, patient habitus, user experience, and so forth) can limit image acquisition. In instances whereby image acquisition is difficult, the parasternal long view can be used to estimate LVEF. For example, if the anterior mitral leaflet fails to come within 1 cm of the ventricular septum in this view, this suggests an EF less than 40% with a sensitivity 69% and specificity of 91%.[26]

As with LV function, assessments of RV systolic function rely on qualitative assessments based on multiple views as well as the demonstration of RV enlargement (which is defined as an RV to LV size ratio >1).[27] Assessments of RV systolic function have been traditionally used to rule in acute pulmonary embolism (PE) or acute coronary syndrome. However, several chronic disease states (eg, dilated cardiomyopathy or pulmonary hypertension) can lead to RV enlargement and can make acute point-of-care assessments challenging. The sensitivity and specificity of RV enlargement or reduced RV systolic function to diagnose PE are low (29% and 51%, respectively).[27] Furthermore, there is only fair to moderate interobserver agreement for RV enlargement and reduced systolic function among certified cardiologists.[28] For these reasons, the American College of Cardiology and the American Society of Echocardiography conclude that the absence of these findings should not be used to rule out PE.[27]

Pericardium

Point-of-care ultrasound can be used to rapidly rule out pericardial effusions in patients with hypotension, which can be particularly helpful because the traditional physician examination findings of pericardial tamponade (eg, Beck triad, pulsus paradoxus) are not present in all patients or have low interobserver agreement.[29] Users can readily detect the presence of pericardial effusions as small as 15 mL with high sensitivity.[30] However, although the absence of a pericardial effusion can help triage critically ill patients, it is more challenging to determine if an effusion is hemodynamically significant with bedside echocardiography. Traditional findings, such as ventricular or atrial collapse, may be present with a sensitivity as low as 50%, whereas inferior vena cava (IVC) dilation is sensitive (97%) but not specific (40%).[30] More formalized assessments for tamponade, such as tricuspid or mitral valve inflow variation, as well as assessments of constrictive pericardial disease are best reserved for a formal echocardiogram.

ASSESSMENT OF VOLUME STATUS

Physical examination maneuvers that assess volume status (eg, jugular venous distension, skin turgor, venous collapse, and so forth) lack sensitivity and interobserver reliability.[31] For example, jugular venous distension has a sensitivity of 39% for acute decompensated heart failure.[31] A key use of bedside echocardiography is the noninvasive assessment of central venous pressure (CVP). Several protocols have been designed to incorporate CVP assessments, including the extended-FAST (E-FAST) scan, rapid ultrasound in shock and hypotension (RUSH), and the cardiopulmonary limited ultrasound examination (CLUE). These protocols are discussed in further detail later. In addition, individualized examinations of the IVC or internal jugular vein (IJV) can be used to guide clinical judgment regarding CVP and the likelihood of fluid responsiveness.

Comprehensive Volume Assessment

Bedside ultrasound has an established role in patients presenting with shock or hypotension, when rapid assessments of CVP are needed. There are now more than 6 protocols that can be performed in patients with cardiac arrest or shock.[32] Perhaps the best known are the E-FAST and RUSH examinations, which are used by emergency and critical care physicians to evaluate hypotension. The RUSH examination components can be remembered with the mnemonic HI-MAP: heart (including the 4 standard transthoracic views), IVC, Morrison pouch, abdominal aorta, and pneumothorax. It has a 97% negative predictive value at ruling out obstructive, hypovolemic, and cardiogenic shock with modest (k = 0.71) interobserver agreement.[33]

The CLUE is a standardized protocol that can elucidate LV function, left atrial enlargement, IVC enlargement, and evidence of pulmonary edema on ultrasonography in the form of comet tails (also known as B-lines) in patients with suspected elevated CVP. The examination and its components have demonstrated moderate to excellent sensitivity, sensitivity, and interobserver reliability for volume overload; a positive test has been shown to be predictive of worsened odds of in-hospital mortality.[34,35]

Inferior Vena Cava

The IVC can be used to estimate CVP based on the vessel's diameter and collapsibility with respiration.[36] It is best measured in the subcostal view approximately 1 to 2 cm from the right atrial junction.[27] Studies investigating the accuracy and interobserver reliability of IVC measurements have varied. For example, resident physicians have moderate interobserver reliability at estimating IVC diameter ($\kappa = 0.60$).[37] IVC imaging should not replace the clinical assessment of volume status and should be incorporated into a more comprehensive clinical assessment.

Internal Jugular Vein

If the IVC cannot be visualized, the IJV provides an alternative method to measure CVP. Several methods exist to estimate CVP based on the IJV, including qualitative assessments based on sonographic wave patterns or measurements of the tissue pressure required to occlude the IJV.[38,39] The Lipton method estimates CVP based on sonographic wave patterns and has a sensitivity/specificity of 98% and 59%, respectively, for an elevated CVP.[40] The use of IJV collapsibility to measure CVP is comparable with the physical examination, although junior trainees may have higher accuracy with handheld ultrasound compared with the physical examination.[41]

ASCITES

Physical examination maneuvers aimed at identifying ascites (eg, shifting dullness or fluid wave detection) may have a sensitivity of 50% to 60% and are limited by patient mobility and body habitus.[42] Point-of-care ultrasound can readily detect ascites with a sensitivity/specificity of 96% and 82%, respectively, with a high concordance with a formal abdominal ultrasound study (k = 0.78).[43] Ultrasound can detect as little as

150 mL of fluid.[44] Even pocket ultrasound devices have 95.8% sensitivity and 81.8% specificity for detecting ascites, and these results are concordant with formal abdominal ultrasounds ($R^2 = 0.781$).[43]

RENAL ULTRASOUND

Point-of-care renal ultrasound can be used by physicians to evaluate patients with acute renal failure or suspected obstructive nephrolithiasis. Although formal ultrasound has a poor sensitivity at detecting renal stones,[45] the presence of hydronephrosis on bedside ultrasound in patients with suspected renal colic can be suggestive of nephrolithiasis[46] and has a pooled sensitivity of 72% to 97% and specificity of 73% to 83% when compared with helical CT in patients with confirmed hydronephrosis due to nephrolithiasis.[46,47] The early use of point-of-care ultrasound in patients with renal colic can reduce emergency department length of stay without a significant increase in secondary visits.[48] This result is likely accomplished through the reduced need for CT scanning if no clinically significant hydronephrosis is present.[48] The ability to detect hydronephrosis via point-of-care ultrasound can be taught to even junior learners with minimal training.[49]

BEYOND POINT-OF-CARE ULTRASOUND: HOW TECHNOLOGY WILL CONTINUE TO SHAPE THE BEDSIDE ENCOUNTER

This limited review of the scope and evidence for the utility of point-of-care ultrasound points to a more extensive adoption of this technology in the future. As machines become smaller, cheaper, and more feature filled, we can expect to see point-of-care ultrasound devices become as ubiquitous as stethoscopes are today. The same technological advances that are making these ultrasound devices smaller and cheaper will create new opportunities for technology to make its way into the bedside encounter. These new technologies will have the same ability to both strengthen and enhance the patient-physician relationship or degrade that relationship depending on how they are used.

A great example of how emerging technology can potentially enhance the patient-physician relationship is virtual medical scribes. Medical scribes have been around for years (often in emergency departments, primary care, and specialty clinics) to decrease the burden of documentation and increase physician efficiency. In the traditional model, a scribe accompanies the physician during a visit to take notes or directly chart into the medical record. Virtual scribes leverage technology to transmit an audio or audio/video feed of the visit to a remote site, where scribes enter the visit notes into the EHR. The promise of this technology is in physician productivity gains but also in allowing the physician to devote greater attention to patients without the distraction of attempting to chart simultaneously.[50] When done well, the technology is barely visible and does not distract from the patient visit, thus, enhancing the experience for both the physician and patients.

Some traditional medical tools are being upgraded by technology. Electronic stethoscopes have existed for decades. They have generally offered sound amplification and occasionally storage as their main features. For physicians with hearing impairment, this sound amplification represented an important feature that allowed them to overcome a disability. Newer devices have additional features, such as friction dampening, ambient noise reduction, and the ability to send the sounds to a cell phone for capture. Electronic stethoscopes allow for recording audio files for teaching. They can also connect to a speaker for improved bedside teaching[3] and to allow patients to listen to their own heart sounds. In the near future, computer algorithms will enhance the diagnostic value of cardiac auscultation by giving physicians an interpretation of the heart sounds much like modern electrocardiogram machines do today.[51]

The challenge of technology for many physicians is adapting to a change in practice and workflow once their formal training is complete. Learning new skills, especially point-of-care ultrasound, is difficult because of the time it takes to learn but also because each physician must decide when they are ready to incorporate the new data into their decision-making process. Continuing medical education courses are available to learn point-of-care ultrasound; however, the training is generally done with healthy volunteers and lacks the clinical context of a patient encounter. Nevertheless, an introductory course is necessary to get started but should be followed by access to a device so that regular practice can occur before incorporation into clinical decision-making.

SUMMARY

Technology's impact on the practice of medicine is sure to continue in the future. New and unforeseen advances are likely and welcome. Like point-of-care ultrasound, each new advance has the opportunity to improve care and potentially improve the patient and physician experience. It is the responsibility of all providers to work to integrate technology into the medical system in a way that enhances patient value and strengthens the patient-physician relationship.

REFERENCES

1. The cost of a cure: revisiting Medicare part D and hepatitis C drugs. Health affairs. Available at: http://healthaffairs.org/blog/2016/11/03/the-cost-of-a-cure-revisiting-medicare-part-d-and-hepatitis-c-drugs/. Accessed June 30, 2017.
2. Verghese A, Charlton B, Cotter B, et al. A history of physical examination texts and the conception of bedside diagnosis. Trans Am Clin Climatol Assoc 2011; 122:290–311.
3. Edelman ER, Weber BN. Tenuous tether. N Engl J Med 2015;373(23):2199–201.
4. Block L, Habicht R, Wu AW, et al. In the wake of the 2003 and 2011 duty hours regulations, how do internal medicine interns spend their time? J Gen Intern Med 2013;28(8):1042–7.
5. Ouyang D, Chen JH, Hom J, et al. Internal medicine resident computer usage: an electronic audit of an inpatient service. JAMA Intern Med 2016;176(2):252–4.
6. Chi J, Verghese A. Clinical education and the electronic health record: the flipped patient. JAMA 2014;312(22):2331–2.
7. Verghese A. Culture shock–patient as icon, icon as patient. N Engl J Med 2008; 359(26):2748–51.
8. Czernik Z, Lin CT. A piece of my mind. Time at the bedside (computing). JAMA 2016;315(22):2399–400.
9. Fleischmann R, Duhm J, Hupperts H, et al. Tablet computers with mobile electronic medical records enhance clinical routine and promote bedside time: a controlled prospective crossover study. J Neurol 2015;262(3):532–40.
10. Moore CL, Copel JA. Point-of-care ultrasonography. N Engl J Med 2011;364(8): 749–57.
11. McKenney M, Lentz K, Nunez D, et al. Can ultrasound replace diagnostic peritoneal lavage in the assessment of blunt trauma? J Trauma 1994;37(3):439–41.
12. Friese RS, Malekzadeh S, Shafi S, et al. Abdominal ultrasound is an unreliable modality for the detection of hemoperitoneum in patients with pelvic fracture. J Trauma 2007;63(1):97–102.
13. Miller MT, Pasquale MD, Bromberg WJ, et al. Not so FAST. J Trauma 2003;54(1): 52–9 [discussion: 59–60].

14. McGahan JP, Rose J, Coates TL, et al. Use of ultrasonography in the patient with acute abdominal trauma. J Ultrasound Med 1997;16(10):653–62 [quiz: 663–4].

15. Nishijima DK, Simel DL, Wisner DH, et al. Does this adult patient have a blunt intra-abdominal injury? JAMA 2012;307(14):1517–27.

16. Evidence report/technology assessment number 43-making health care safer: a critical analysis of patient safety practices. Available at: https://archive.ahrq.gov/clinic/ptsafety/pdf/ptsafety.pdf.

17. Guidance on the use of ultrasound locating devices for placing central venous catheters | guidance and guidelines | NICE. Available at: https://www.nice.org.uk/guidance/ta49. Accessed July 30, 2017.

18. Gordon CE, Feller-Kopman D, Balk EM, et al. Pneumothorax following thoracentesis: a systematic review and meta-analysis. Arch Intern Med 2010;170(4):332–9.

19. Mercaldi CJ, Lanes SF. Ultrasound guidance decreases complications and improves the cost of care among patients undergoing thoracentesis and paracentesis. Chest 2013;143(2):532–8.

20. Aponte H, Acosta S, Rigamonti D, et al. The use of ultrasound for placement of intravenous catheters. AANA J 2007;75(3):212–6.

21. Shokoohi H, Boniface K, McCarthy M, et al. Ultrasound-guided peripheral intravenous access program is associated with a marked reduction in central venous catheter use in noncritically ill emergency department patients. Ann Emerg Med 2013;61(2):198–203.

22. Levitov A, Frankel HL, Blaivas M, et al. Guidelines for the appropriate use of bedside general and cardiac ultrasonography in the evaluation of critically ill patients—part II: cardiac ultrasonography. Crit Care Med 2016;44(6):1206.

23. Ultrasound policy 2016 complete.pdf.

24. Spencer KT, Kimura BJ, Korcarz CE, et al. Focused cardiac ultrasound: recommendations from the American Society of Echocardiography. J Am Soc Echocardiogr 2013;26(6):567–81.

25. Razi R, Estrada JR, Doll J, et al. Bedside hand-carried ultrasound by internal medicine residents versus traditional clinical assessment for the identification of systolic dysfunction in patients admitted with decompensated heart failure. J Am Soc Echocardiogr 2011;24(12):1319–24.

26. Kimura BJ, Shaw DJ, Amundson SA, et al. Cardiac limited ultrasound examination techniques to augment the bedside cardiac physical examination. J Ultrasound Med 2015;34(9):1683–90.

27. Labovitz AJ, Noble VE, Bierig M, et al. Focused cardiac ultrasound in the emergent setting: a consensus statement of the American Society of Echocardiography and American College of Emergency Physicians. J Am Soc Echocardiogr 2010;23(12):1225–30.

28. Kopecna D, Briongos S, Castillo H, et al. Interobserver reliability of echocardiography for prognostication of normotensive patients with pulmonary embolism. Cardiovasc Ultrasound 2014;12:29.

29. Roy CL, Minor MA, Brookhart MA, et al. Does this patient with a pericardial effusion have cardiac tamponade? JAMA 2007;297(16):1810–8.

30. Ceriani E, Cogliati C. Update on bedside ultrasound diagnosis of pericardial effusion. Intern Emerg Med 2016;11(3):477–80.

31. Wang CS, FitzGerald JM, Schulzer M, et al. Does this dyspneic patient in the emergency department have congestive heart failure? JAMA 2005;294(15):1944–56.

32. Peterson D, Arntfield RT. Critical care ultrasonography. Emerg Med Clin North Am 2014;32(4):907–26.

33. Ghane MR, Gharib MH, Ebrahimi A, et al. Accuracy of rapid ultrasound in shock (RUSH) exam for diagnosis of shock in critically ill patients. Trauma Mon 2015; 20(1):e20095.
34. Gottlieb M, Bailitz J. What is the clinical utility of bedside ultrasonography in the diagnosis of acute cardiogenic pulmonary edema in the undifferentiated dyspneic patient? Ann Emerg Med 2015;66(3):283–4.
35. Randazzo MR, Snoey ER, Levitt MA, et al. Accuracy of emergency physician assessment of left ventricular ejection fraction and central venous pressure using echocardiography. Acad Emerg Med 2003;10(9):973–7.
36. Rudski LG, Lai WW, Afilalo J, et al. Guidelines for the echocardiographic assessment of the right heart in adults: a report from the American Society of Echocardiography endorsed by the European Association of Echocardiography, a registered branch of the European Society of Cardiology, and the Canadian Society of Echocardiography. J Am Soc Echocardiogr 2010;23(7):685–713 [quiz: 786–8].
37. Akkaya A, Yesilaras M, Aksay E, et al. The interrater reliability of ultrasound imaging of the inferior vena cava performed by emergency residents. Am J Emerg Med 2013;31(10):1509–11.
38. Baumann UA, Marquis C, Stoupis C, et al. Estimation of central venous pressure by ultrasound. Resuscitation 2005;64(2):193–9.
39. Lipton B. Estimation of central venous pressure by ultrasound of the internal jugular vein. Am J Emerg Med 2000;18(4):432–4.
40. Jang T, Aubin C, Naunheim R, et al. Jugular venous distension on ultrasound: sensitivity and specificity for heart failure in patients with dyspnea. Am J Emerg Med 2011;29(9):1198–202.
41. Rizkallah J, Jack M, Saeed M, et al. Non-invasive bedside assessment of central venous pressure: scanning into the future. PLoS One 2014;9(10):e109215.
42. Williams JW Jr, Simel DL. The rational clinical examination. Does this patient have ascites? How to divine fluid in the abdomen. JAMA 1992;267(19):2645–8.
43. Keil-Ríos D, Terrazas-Solís H, González-Garay A, et al. Pocket ultrasound device as a complement to physical examination for ascites evaluation and guided paracentesis. Intern Emerg Med 2016;11(3):461–6.
44. Von Kuenssberg Jehle D, Stiller G, Wagner D. Sensitivity in detecting free intraperitoneal fluid with the pelvic views of the FAST exam. Am J Emerg Med 2003; 21(6):476–8.
45. Dickman E, Tessaro MO, Arroyo AC, et al. Clinician-performed abdominal sonography. Eur J Trauma Emerg Surg 2015;41(5):481–92.
46. Dalziel PJ, Noble VE. Bedside ultrasound and the assessment of renal colic: a review. Emerg Med J 2013;30(1):3–8.
47. Riddell J, Case A, Wopat R, et al. Sensitivity of emergency bedside ultrasound to detect hydronephrosis in patients with computed tomography-proven stones. West J Emerg Med 2014;15(1):96–100.
48. Park YH, Jung RB, Lee YG, et al. Does the use of bedside ultrasonography reduce emergency department length of stay for patients with renal colic?: a pilot study. Clin Exp Emerg Med 2016;3(4):197–203.
49. Mandavia DP, Aragona J, Chan L, et al. Ultrasound training for emergency physicians–a prospective study. Acad Emerg Med 2000;7(9):1008–14.
50. Brady K, Shariff A. Virtual medical scribes: making electronic medical records work for you. J Med Pract Manage 2013;29(2):133–6.
51. Leng S, Tan RS, Chai KTC, et al. The electronic stethoscope. Biomed Eng Online 2015;14:66.

Diagnostic Errors and the Bedside Clinical Examination

Bennett W. Clark, MD[a],*, Arsalan Derakhshan, MD[a],
Sanjay V. Desai, MD[b]

KEYWORDS

- Diagnostic error • Clinical reasoning • Clinical decision-making
- Heuristics and biases • Dual-processing theory • Medical education

KEY POINTS

- Diagnostic errors are common in clinical practice and result in adverse patient outcomes.
- Diagnostic errors are frequently unrecognized and under-reported because of individual and systematic factors.
- Deficiencies or omissions in the bedside clinical examination and in disease-specific content knowledge are among the most common causes of diagnostic errors.
- Unconscious heuristics and biases contribute to diagnostic errors.
- Research in clinical settings suggests that education in clinical content knowledge and bedside history and physical examination skills can reduce diagnostic errors.

INTRODUCTION

In 2014, a 48-year-old woman with a history of stroke and uncontrolled diabetes presented to her local hospital for evaluation of a lesion on the left side of her face (**Fig. 1**). Previous swabs of the lesion had grown methicillin-resistant *Staphylococcus aureus*, so her doctors diagnosed her with cellulitis and sent her home with a peripherally inserted central catheter (PICC) line and a 10-day course of intravenous (IV) vancomycin. Unfortunately, the lesion did not improve, and she returned to the same hospital

Disclosure: The authors certify that they have no affiliations with or involvement in any organization or entity with any financial interest (ie, honoraria; educational grants; participation in speakers' bureaus; membership, employment, consultancies, stock ownership, or other equity interest; and expert testimony or patent-licensing arrangements), or nonfinancial interest (ie, personal or professional relationships, affiliations, knowledge or beliefs) in the subject matter or materials discussed in this article.

[a] Department of Internal Medicine, Johns Hopkins University School of Medicine, 600 North Wolfe Street, Baltimore, MD 21287, USA; [b] Department of Internal Medicine, Johns Hopkins University School of Medicine, 1830 East Monument Street, Baltimore, MD 21287, USA
* Corresponding author. Department of Internal Medicine, University of Minnesota School of Medicine, 420 Delaware Street Southeast, MMC 741, Minneapolis, MN 55455.
E-mail address: Bclark@umn.edu

Med Clin N Am 102 (2018) 453–464
https://doi.org/10.1016/j.mcna.2017.12.007
medical.theclinics.com

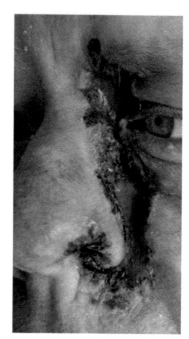

Fig. 1. 48-year-old woman with trigeminal trophic syndrome.

twice over the next year. Both times, her doctors sent her home with a PICC line for more IV vancomycin. Convinced that the woman had refractory cellulitis, her outpatient doctors gave her additional courses of oral antibiotics. Despite these treatments, the lesion on her face never improved.

More than a year later, she was admitted to the general medicine service of a teaching hospital. Her neurologic examination revealed decreased sensation on the right side of her body and a left-sided Horner syndrome consistent with a prior lateral medullary stroke, a diagnosis confirmed by review of a prior MRI scan. Additionally, a punch biopsy of the facial lesion showed no evidence of cancer, infection, or autoimmune pathology. This, combined with evidence of injury to the left spinal trigeminal nucleus led to the diagnosis of trigeminal trophic syndrome—a rare, noninfectious condition caused by neuropathic itch, decreased facial sensation, and chronic skin abrasion from scratching in the distribution of the trigeminal nerve.[1]

In the end, it took more than a year to give the woman an accurate diagnosis. Why did it take so long, and what explains the tenacity of the cellulitis diagnosis despite abundant evidence against it? Finally, and most importantly, how can it be done better?

Diagnostic error is a central concern in medicine and has had increased focus from stakeholders across the professional community and the public over the last 20 years. This article aims to orient readers to this complex field, with particular attention to

1. The impact of diagnostic errors on patient outcomes
2. Controversies in defining and studying diagnostic errors
3. Diagnostic errors common in clinical practice
4. Conditions, both environmental and cognitive, that predispose doctors to making diagnostic errors
5. Methods for improving diagnostic accuracy

THE IMPACT OF DIAGNOSTIC ERRORS ON PATIENT OUTCOMES

Diagnosis is at the heart of a doctor's craft. It is the precondition of effective treatment and the foundation of trust between doctor and patient.[2] It is also a point of professional pride. When doctors realize they have missed a diagnosis, they feel guilt and remorse.[3]

But diagnostic errors take a far greater toll on patients' lives than on doctors' psyches. "To Err is Human," a landmark study published by the Institute of Medicine (IOM) in 1999, estimated that diagnostic errors were responsible for 17% of preventable adverse hospital events.[4] A review of more than 30,000 New York hospital records found that 14% of hospital errors were diagnostic in nature, and that most diagnostic errors were not only preventable but negligent.[5] The problem is no less serious in the outpatient setting. Observational studies suggest that primary care doctors miss about 12 million diagnoses each year, and that about half of these misses cause patients significant harm.[6]

Advanced medical technology appears to make only a marginal impact on diagnostic accuracy. Studies comparing the frequency of missed diagnoses before and after the advent of modern diagnostic imaging found little improvement in diagnostic accuracy.[7,8] A more recent analysis[9] argues that this lack of improvement is likely an artifact of clinical selection bias. Autopsies are far less common than they were prior to the use of cross-sectional imaging, and cases that do proceed to autopsy tend to be complex. Controlling for this selection bias, the rate of major diagnostic error is likely around 8%, in line with recent reviews of intensive care unit (ICU) autopsy cases. Even at this modestly improved error rate, as many as 35,000 patients die in US hospitals each year because of a missed diagnosis.[10,11]

CONTROVERSIES IN DEFINING AND STUDYING DIAGNOSTIC ERRORS

Diagnosis can refer to the explanation for a patient's condition, or the process of arriving at this explanation. This ambiguity has contributed to a lack of systematicity in research on diagnostic error. Newman-Toker helped resolve these semantic problems by distinguishing between failures in the diagnostic process and failures in diagnostic labeling[12] (**Fig. 2**). Most clinicians can easily recall cases in which these 2 types of error were linked, when flawed thinking led to an incorrect or delayed diagnosis. However, it is also possible to get the process wrong but the label right, such as when a radiologist misses a malignant tumor on chest radiograph, but the cancer is

Diagnostic Label

		Accurate	Inaccurate
Diagnostic Process	Sound	True Diagnosis	Unavoidable Diagnostic Error
	Unsound	Near Miss	Avoidable Diagnostic Error

Fig. 2. Schema for the classification of diagnostic errors. (*Data from* Newman-Toker DE. A unified conceptual model for diagnostic errors: underdiagnosis, overdiagnosis, and misdiagnosis. Diagnosis (Berl) 2014;1(1):43–8.)

identified by another member of the health care team before the malignancy progresses in stage.[10] In this case, the patient receives the correct label despite a flaw in the process. In Newman-Toker's updated taxonomy of diagnostic errors, these instances of flawed diagnostic reasoning leading to an accurate diagnostic label are called near misses.[13]

The reverse can also happen. Kassirer and Kopelman described a 53-year-old woman who returned from an overseas trip during which she had eaten at unsanitary restaurants and developed diarrhea. Microscopic examination of her stool revealed multiple parasites, and she was diagnosed with intestinal parasitosis. However, her diarrhea worsened after treatment for parasites, and she was ultimately diagnosed with a vasoactive intestinal peptide (VIP)-secreting tumor.[7] Newman-Toker calls these cases, along with conditions that cannot be diagnosed using current medical technology, as unavoidable diagnostic errors. Although this is an important conceptual distinction, the practicing clinician may wonder, justifiably, whether something unavoidable should be considered an error at all. In keeping with the preponderance of current research on diagnostic error, this article focuses on avoidable errors.

DIAGNOSTIC ERRORS COMMON IN CLINICAL PRACTICE
Diagnosis Label Failures

Doctors have limited insight into their diagnostic skills.[8,13] They have similar confidence with common, standardized clinical cases, which they diagnose correctly more than half of the time, as with unusual cases, which they solve correctly only 5% of the time.[14] A retrospective review of autopsy cases from a medical intensive care unit found that doctors who were completely certain of their diagnosis were wrong 40% of the time.[15] Overconfidence is not unique to the medical profession, and examples of this better-than-average effect are widely reported in social psychology literature.[16] Put simply, without external feedback, doctors rarely predict the accuracy of their diagnoses. This phenomenon is reflected in reviews of error-reporting systems, in which computerized error identification turns up 10 times as many errors as physician self-report.[17]

Individualized data on diagnostic error are lacking, so most information on missed diagnoses often comes from pooled data sets. For example, missed cases of cancer account for more than half of malpractice claims against outpatient internal medicine physicians.[18] Singh and colleagues[19] performed a retrospective review of 209 missed diagnoses in the ambulatory setting, in which the most common missed diagnosis was pneumonia, at 7% of the total. Missed primary cancer accounted for 6% of the total missed diagnoses in this study. Voluntary surveys of doctors, which are susceptible to recall biases, report primary cancers as the most common category of missed diagnosis,[20,21] highlighting the challenge of measuring the rates of diagnostic errors accurately.

Diagnostic Process Failures

Failures in diagnostic processing and clinical reasoning are more difficult to identify than failures in diagnostic labeling. Advances in cognitive psychology over the last 50 years have uncovered some of the reasons why, beginning with the fact that, as doctors gain experience, they rely heavily on rapid, unconscious processes to make diagnoses.[22] Thus, the specific processes a doctor uses to arrive at a diagnosis are hidden not only from researchers but also from the doctor. Even when doctors take the artificial step of thinking aloud about their diagnostic process, their descriptions are unreliable.[23] Moreover, once doctors or other observers know the outcome of a case, they consistently overestimate what could have been known prior to the diagnosis being firmly established, a phenomenon known as hindsight bias.[24]

Useful frameworks to examine the features and failures in diagnostic processing have been developed (**Fig. 3**). Kassirer and Kopelman divided the process into 4 steps:

1. Hypothesis generation, which they called triggering
2. Framing the patient's problem
3. Gathering and processing information, such as findings on the clinical examination and laboratory tests
4. Verifying the diagnosis by making sure that competing hypotheses can be reasonably excluded

They found that errors in gathering and processing information were the most common, followed by errors in triggering.[16]

SYSTEMS, COGNITIVE AND PRACTICE-RELATED CONTRIBUTIONS TO DIAGNOSTIC ERROR
System-Related Factors

Organizational and environmental factors play an important role in diagnostic errors. Among these factors are

- Reimbursement structures that discourage consultation
- Incomplete medical records
- Cultural and logistical barriers to communication between doctors
- High physician workloads
- Patient failure to follow up
- Community hospital settings (compared with teaching hospitals)[25]

Cognitive Factors

Heuristics are methods used to solve problems quickly. Doctors use heuristics to make diagnoses all the time. However, heuristics can also lead to errors, because they can introduce unconscious biases. In the early 1970s, the cognitive psychologists Amos Tversky and Daniel Kahneman demonstrated that heuristics lead to predictable errors in judgment. In 1 experiment, they played a tape-recorded list of names, then asked participants to estimate whether the list included more women or men. When

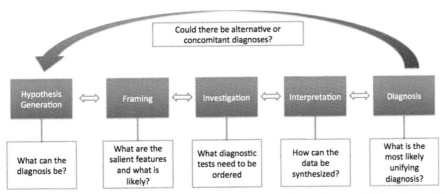

Fig. 3. Conceptual map of the diagnostic process. (*Data from* Kassirer JP, Kopelman RI. Cognitive errors in diagnosis: instantiation, classification, and consequences. Am J Med 1989;86(4):433–41.)

the list included famous women (eg, Elizabeth Taylor) and less famous men (eg, William Fulbright), 80% of participants erroneously believed the list had more women.[26] This phenomenon of overestimating the frequency of things that come to mind readily is now called availability bias.

Heuristics and their associated biases have been subsumed into an overarching model of cognitive reasoning called dual-processing theory. This theory describes 2 systems for making judgments and decisions. System 1 is rapid, instinctive, automatic, and driven by networks of associations. Take a moment to look at the face in **Fig. 4**. After just a few seconds, you will have made numerous inferences about the person's age, mood, and background. These rapid judgments represent the outcome of System 1 processing. System 2, on the other hand, is deliberate, sequential, logical, and demands cognitive energy. Try to solve the following problem without pen or paper: 673 x 779. To have any chance of success, one must block out distractions and come up with a plan for keeping track of multiplied values. This is a System 2 task.[27] Not surprisingly, physicians rely more heavily on System 1 as they become more experienced.[28]

Croskerry has described how patterns of bias can corrupt diagnostic reasoning. His survey[29] of 32 common errors in diagnostic reasoning includes habits of thought that most doctors will find familiar, such as the sunk costs phenomenon—"the more clinicians invest in a particular diagnosis, the less likely they may be to release it and consider alternatives"—and anchoring—"the tendency to perceptually lock onto salient features in the patient's initial presentation too early in the diagnostic process, failing to adjust this initial impression in light of later information." An abbreviated version of Croskerry's list is presented in **Table 1**.

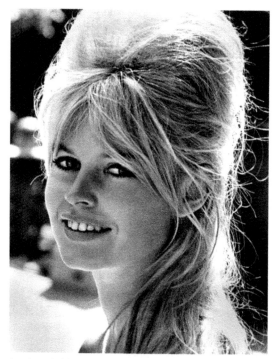

Fig. 4. Brigitte Bardot.(*Available* via Wikimedia Commons: https://commons.wikimedia.org/wiki/File:Brigitte_Bardot_-_1962.jpg. Accessed June 8, 2017.)

Table 1 Common biases that lead to diagnostic errors	
Aggregate bias	The tendency to believe that aggregated data, such as those used to develop clinical practice guidelines, do not apply to individual patients (especially their own)
Anchoring	The tendency to perceptually lock onto salient features in the patient's initial presentation too early in the diagnostic process failing to adjust this initial impression in the light of later information; this CDR may be severely compounded by the confirmation bias
Availability bias	The disposition to judge things as being more likely, or frequently occurring, if they readily come to mind; recent experience with a disease may inflate the likelihood of its being diagnosed, and conversely, if a disease has not been seen for a long time (is less available), it may be underdiagnosed
Confirmation bias	The tendency to look for confirming evidence to support a diagnosis rather than look for disconfirming evidence to refute it, despite the latter often being more persuasive and definitive
Outcome bias	The tendency to opt for diagnostic decisions that will lead to good outcomes, rather than those associated with bad outcomes, thereby avoiding chagrin associated with the latter
Overconfidence bias	A universal tendency to believe one knows more than he or she does; overconfidence reflects a tendency to act on incomplete information, intuitions, or hunches
Premature closure	The tendency to apply premature closure to the decision-making process, accepting a diagnosis before it has been fully verified
Psych-out error:	The tendency to attribute presenting symptoms to psychiatric etiologies, especially in patients carrying a psychiatric diagnosis; serious medical conditions can be misdiagnosed as psychiatric conditions
Representative restraint	The tendency to look for prototypical manifestations of disease, which leads to atypical variants being missed

Adapted from Croskerry P. The importance of cognitive errors in diagnosis and strategies to minimize them. Acad Med 2003;78(8):777–8; with permission.

Although many writers and researchers have described these flawed decision processes, few have undertaken rigorous studies of how they influence patient care. Researchers in the Netherlands have demonstrated the power of availability bias in skewing clinical cases presented to trainees in a booklet.[30,31] A prospective study of trainees managing simulated emergencies found that premature closure (31%) and confirmation bias (30%) were the most common cognitive contributors to erroneous diagnosis.[32] By contrast, a prospective analysis by Voytovich of student and physician efforts to solve 3 written clinical cases found that more than 90% of participants missed a diagnosis because of premature closure.[33] To the authors' knowledge, no prospective studies have examined cognitive bias in patient care environments.

The discrepancies in these studies' findings reflects a general lack of standardization among researchers investigating the cognitive psychology of diagnosis. Did Voytovich's study differ from the study of simulated emergencies because it was conducted in a different setting, because of different methods for obtaining data about participants clinical reasoning, or because of different definitions of what counts as premature closure? The current literature on the cognitive psychology of clinical diagnosis is not mature enough to answer these questions.

Some psychologists, postulating that heuristics are hardwired into the decision-making process by evolution, argue that the biases described are difficult if not impossible to unlearn. Others have attempted to show that reminding physicians about their biases and fallibility is a promising way to reduce diagnostic error. These efforts are described in the next section under the heading Reflective Practice.

The Missing Bedside Examination

When doctors recall cases in which they missed a diagnosis, they frequently report performing an incomplete bedside examination.[34] Association between faulty bedside assessment and diagnostic error is corroborated in a systematic review of medical malpractice cases, in which failure to perform an adequate history and physical examination contributed to 42% of missed diagnoses. The same review showed almost 70% of missed cancer cases were because of an inadequate history and physical examination.[34] In reviews of computer-identified diagnostic errors in outpatient internal medicine clinics, more than half of cases involved a shortcoming in the history or physical examination.[26]

Disease-specific studies examining trends in missed diagnoses among grave conditions with benign mimics suggest that deficiencies in bedside clinical evaluation often contribute to diagnostic delay. A retrospective review of cases of ruptured aortic abdominal aneurysm (AAA) found that doctors missed this diagnosis 61% of the time. Unfamiliarity with the cardinal signs of a contained AAA rupture—urinary retention, flank pain, abdominal distension, leukocytosis, and an absence of shock or anemia—was common among doctors missing the diagnosis, as was a failure to palpate large AAAs, even in patients without abdominal distension.[35] Kowalski and colleagues[36] reviewed 56 cases of missed subarachnoid hemorrhage and found that doctors' unfamiliarity with the phenomenon of sentinel headaches correlated with missed diagnosis.

Clinical mimicry, combined with deficiencies in the clinical examination, also contributes to overdiagnosis. A retrospective review of patients referred to a Lyme disease specialty clinic found that 77% did not have active Lyme disease, and that many patients would have avoided misdiagnosis if their referring physicians had been able to distinguish degenerative arthritis from Lyme arthritis.[37]

HOW TO IMPROVE DIAGNOSTIC ACCURACY
System-Based Interventions

The literature examining real-world methods for avoiding diagnostic error is limited, especially in light of the abundant theoretic writing on the topic in the past decade. Although data are sparse, experts are optimistic about electronic medical records' (EMRs) ability to reduce errors, not only by catching them before they become clinically consequential, but also by actively steering clinicians toward accurate diagnoses.[38] Nonrandomized prospective studies have demonstrated effectiveness of electronic interventions using several approaches:

- A diagnostic decision support system (DDSS) that generated diagnostic suggestions based on preliminary clinical data improved the accuracy of pediatrics reisdents.[39]
- Computer-guided patient histories can provide important clinical data that physicians fail to elicit.[40]
- An automated electrocardiogram (ECG) interpretation program improved interns' accuracy in the diagnosis of acute myocardial ischemia.[41]

The most common system-based intervention aimed at enhancing patient out-comes by reducing diagnostic error involves building redundancy into the interpreta-tion of diagnostic tests.[42] Redundancy is especially relevant for clinical pathology and radiology, where data suggest that interpretation of a study by more than 1 physician can improve test sensitivity. For example, review of computed tomography (CT) colo-noscopies by 2 radiologists instead of one increased sensitivity for underlying colon cancer, although it also decreased specificity.[43] Although such strict methods of redundancy may not seem relevant for internal medicine, Graber and colleagues[44] note that the impulse to seek help from colleagues, whether through curbside consul-tation or a formal second opinion, can also improve diagnostic accuracy, a premise that has been confirmed in simulated clinical problem solving.[45]

Reflective Practice

Cognitive psychologists spent much of the twentieth century cataloging System 1's habitual inaccuracy,[38] so it should come as no surprise that much of the current clin-ical reasoning research aims at getting diagnosticians out of System 1 and into Sys-tem 2. The idea is that one can reduce diagnostic error by thinking slow instead of fast.

For example, a group of psychologists in the Netherlands presented internal med-icine residents with a booklet of clinical vignettes that had been selected to activate availability bias, a well-described bias of System 1. Residents who solved the cases in an unstructured manner were less accurate than those who went through a pre-scribed process of listing data for and against their initial diagnosis before deciding on a final diagnosis.[41] A prospective study evaluating undergraduate students' ability to learn ECG interpretation found that they were more accurate when receiving this prompt: "Don't jump the gun; consider the feature list before providing a final diagnosis."[46]

Common sense suggests that a slow, deliberative approach to diagnosis is not needed in all cases. For an experienced clinician, common syndromes with clear signs—decompensated heart failure, cirrhosis, psoriasis—do not require a second thought. A study comparing diagnostic strategies in simple and complex cases sup-ports this premise; for simple cases, deliberation does not boost diagnostic accuracy. For complex cases, it does.[47]

Unfortunately, no pro-System 2 study has been conducted in a clinical setting. The result is research that confirms something most diagnosticians already understand: when posed with cases that are complex, challenging, or misleading, clinicians do a better job when they have the time, space, and resources to slow down and organize their thoughts. The more difficult question is how clinicians can better recognize cases that require a System 2 approach, and how medical technology, workflows, and infra-structure can better support clinicians when such cases arise. Consider the example of the woman at the beginning of this article. For more than a year, her physicians approached her case with a decidedly System 1 approach, diagnosing her over and over with cellulitis. The fact that she had completed multiple courses of IV antibiotics without getting better should have prompted reconsideration of the diagnosis, but it did not. What training could her doctors have received to help them toggle from Sys-tem 1 to System 2? How could their working environment have been improved to help them do so? These are active areas of research for proponents of cognitive debiasing and reflective practice.

The Clinical Examination and Clinical Content Knowledge

Imagine that the patient described previously had been treated by doctors capable of recognizing the signs of a lateral medullary stroke. If they had known what they were looking at in the first place, an effortful System 2 analysis might not have been needed to diagnose trigeminal trophic syndrome. It is also possible that they were able to recognize such signs, but never stopped to look. Reviews of malpractice claims and surveys of physicians suggest that failure to perform a complete bedside examination underlies many diagnostic errors. To correct this failing, 1 expert has recommended that clinicians use a diagnostic checklist, the first 2 steps of which are to obtain a complete history and complete a purposeful physical examination.

Education in bedside medicine has the potential to reduce diagnostic errors. The evidence for such interventions is more robust than the evidence for cognitive debiasing and reflective practice, having been proven in real-world clinical settings. Several prospective studies have demonstrated that provider-specific feedback and disease-specific education improve diagnostic accuracy. Providing emergency room physicians with intensive, real-time feedback on the outcomes of discharged patients decreased physicians' rate of adverse events.[48] Similar interventions with attending psychiatrists and trainees in clinical psychology resulted in improvements in diagnostic accuracy.[49] A regional program to educate primary care physicians on the clinical presentation of subarachnoid hemorrhage resulted in more timely diagnosis for patients with this life-threatening syndrome.[50] A renewed emphasis on the bedside examination and deliberate feedback loops to physicians may be the most effective way to reduce diagnostic errors.

SUMMARY

Diagnostic errors cause patients serious harm. Such errors arise from a complex set of factors at both the system and the clinician level. Although most interventions to reduce diagnostic error have focused on system-level improvements, recent advances in cognitive psychology have prompted debate on how best to improve clinicians' diagnostic reasoning. A limited body of evidence suggests that adjusting habits of thought can lead to more accurate diagnosis. However, the preponderance of evidence in this field points to the importance of improving bedside skills and receiving detailed clinical feedback.

REFERENCES

1. Sawada T, Asai J, Nomiyama T, et al. Trigeminal trophic syndrome: report of a case and review of the published work. J Dermatol 2014;41(6):525–8.
2. Osler W. Aequanimitas. Philadelphia: P Blackiston's Son & Co; 1920.
3. Ely JW, Levinson W, Elder NC, et al. Perceived causes of family physicians' errors. J Fam Pract 1995;40(4):337–44.
4. Kohn LT, Corrigan J, Donaldson MS. To err is human: building a safer health system. Washington, DC: National Academy Press; 2000.
5. Leape LL, Brennan TA, Laird N, et al. The nature of adverse events in hospitalized patients. Results of the Harvard Medical Practice Study II. N Engl J Med 1991; 324(6):377–84.
6. Singh H, Meyer AN, Thomas EJ. The frequency of diagnostic errors in outpatient care: estimations from three large observational studies involving US adult populations. BMJ Qual Saf 2014;23(9):727–31.
7. Goldman L, Sayson R, Robbins S, et al. The value of the autopsy in three medical eras. N Engl J Med 1983;308(17):1000–5.
8. Veress B, Alafuzoff I. A retrospective analysis of clinical diagnoses and autopsy findings in 3,042 cases during two different time periods. Hum Pathol 1994;25(2): 140–5.

9. Shojania KG, Burton EC, McDonald KM, et al. Changes in rates of autopsy-detected diagnostic errors over time: a systematic review. JAMA 2003;289(21): 2849–56.

10. Quekel LG, Kessels AG, Goei R, et al. Miss rate of lung cancer on the chest radiograph in clinical practice. Chest 1999;115(3):720–4.

11. Dhaliwal G. Known unknowns and unknown unknowns at the point of care. JAMA Intern Med 2013;173(21):1959–61.

12. Newman-Toker DE. A unified conceptual model for diagnostic errors: underdiagnosis, overdiagnosis, and misdiagnosis. Diagnosis (Berl) 2014;1(1):43–8.

13. Eva KW, Regehr G. Self-assessment in the health professions: a reformulation and research agenda. Acad Med 2005;80(10 Suppl):S46–54.

14. Meyer AN, Payne VL, Meeks DW, et al. Physicians' diagnostic accuracy, confidence, and resource requests: a vignette study. JAMA Intern Med 2013; 173(21):1952–8.

15. Podbregar M, Voga G, Krivec B, et al. Should we confirm our clinical diagnostic certainty by autopsies? Intensive Care Med 2001;27(11):1750–5.

16. Pronin E, Gilovich T, Ross L. Objectivity in the eye of the beholder: divergent perceptions of bias in self versus others. Psychol Rev 2004;111(3):781–99.

17. Johnson CW. How will we get the data and what will we do with it then? Issues in the reporting of adverse healthcare events. Qual Saf Health Care 2003;12(Suppl 2):ii64–7.

18. Gandhi TK, Kachalia A, Thomas EJ, et al. Missed and delayed diagnoses in the ambulatory setting: a study of closed malpractice claims. Ann Intern Med 2006; 145(7):488–96.

19. Singh H, Giardina TD, Meyer AN, et al. Types and origins of diagnostic errors in primary care settings. JAMA Intern Med 2013;173(6):418–25.

20. Schiff GD, Hasan O, Kim S, et al. Diagnostic error in medicine: analysis of 583 physician-reported errors. Arch Intern Med 2009;169(20):1881–7.

21. Ely JW, Kaldjian LC, D'Alessandro DM. Diagnostic errors in primary care: lessons learned. J Am Board Fam Med 2012;25(1):87–97.

22. Custers EJ, Regehr G, Norman GR. Mental representations of medical diagnostic knowledge: a review. Acad Med 1996;71(10 Suppl):S55–61.

23. Ward M, Gruppen L, Regehr G. Measuring self-assessment: current state of the art. Adv Health Sci Educ Theor Pract 2002;7(1):63–80.

24. Wears RL, Nemeth CP. Replacing hindsight with insight: toward better understanding of diagnostic failures. Ann Emerg Med 2007;49(2):206–9.

25. Sarkar U, Simchowitz B, Bonacum D, et al. A qualitative analysis of physician perspectives on missed and delayed outpatient diagnosis: the focus on system-related factors. Jt Comm J Qual Patient Saf 2014;40(10):461–70.

26. Tversky A, Kahneman D. Availability: a heuristic for judging frequency and probability. Cogn Psychol 1973;5(2):207–32.

27. Kahneman D. Thinking fast and slow. New York: Farrar, Strauss and Giroux; 2011.

28. Schmidt H, Boshuizen H. On acquiring expertise in medicine. Educ Psychol Rev 1993;593:205–21.

29. Croskerry P. The importance of cognitive errors in diagnosis and strategies to minimize them. Acad Med 2003;78(8):775–80.

30. Mamede S, van Gog T, van den Berge K, et al. Effect of availability bias and reflective reasoning on diagnostic accuracy among internal medicine residents. JAMA 2010;304(11):1198–203.

31. Schmidt HG, Mamede S, van den Berge K, et al. Exposure to media information about a disease can cause doctors to misdiagnose similar-looking clinical cases. Acad Med 2014;89(2):285–91.

32. Stiegler MP, Neelankavil JP, Canales C, et al. Cognitive errors detected in anaesthesiology: a literature review and pilot study. Br J Anaesth 2012;108(2):229–35.

33. Voytovich AE, Rippey RM, Suffredini A. Premature conclusions in diagnostic reasoning. J Med Educ 1985;60(4):302–7.

34. Verghese A, Charlton B, Kassirer JP, et al. Inadequacies of physical examination as a cause of medical errors and adverse events: a collection of vignettes. Am J Med 2015;128(12):1322–4.e3.

35. Lederle FA, Parenti CM, Chute EP. Ruptured abdominal aortic aneurysm: the internist as diagnostician. Am J Med 1994;96(2):163–7.

36. Kowalski RG, Claassen J, Kreiter KT, et al. Initial misdiagnosis and outcome after subarachnoid hemorrhage. JAMA 2004;291(7):866–9.

37. Steere AC, Taylor E, McHugh GL, et al. The overdiagnosis of Lyme disease. JAMA 1993;269(14):1812–6.

38. Schiff GD, Bates DW. Can electronic clinical documentation help prevent diagnostic errors? N Engl J Med 2010;362(12):1066–9.

39. Ramnarayan P, Winrow A, Coren M, et al. Diagnostic omission errors in acute paediatric practice: impact of a reminder system on decision-making. BMC Med Inform Decis Mak 2006;6:37.

40. Zakim D, Braun N, Fritz P, et al. Underutilization of information and knowledge in everyday medical practice: evaluation of a computer-based solution. BMC Med Inform Decis Mak 2008;8:50.

41. Olsson SE, Ohlsson M, Ohlin H, et al. Decision support for the initial triage of patients with acute coronary syndromes. Clin Physiol Funct Imaging 2006;26(3): 151–6.

42. McDonald KM, Matesic B, Contopoulos-Ioannidis DG, et al. Patient safety strategies targeted at diagnostic errors: a systematic review. Ann Intern Med 2013; 158(5 Pt 2):381–9.

43. Murphy R, Slater A, Uberoi R, et al. Reduction of perception error by double reporting of minimal preparation CT colon. Br J Radiol 2010;83(988):331–5.

44. Graber ML, Kissam S, Payne VL, et al. Cognitive interventions to reduce diagnostic error: a narrative review. BMJ Qual Saf 2012;21(7):535–57.

45. Christensen C, Larson JR Jr, Abbott A, et al. Decision making of clinical teams: communication patterns and diagnostic error. Med Decis Making 2000;20(1):45–50.

46. Eva KW, Hatala RM, Leblanc VR, et al. Teaching from the clinical reasoning literature: combined reasoning strategies help novice diagnosticians overcome misleading information. Med Educ 2007;41(12):1152–8.

47. Mamede S, Schmidt HG, Rikers RM, et al. Conscious thought beats deliberation without attention in diagnostic decision-making: at least when you are an expert. Psychol Res 2010;74(6):586–92.

48. Chern CH, How CK, Wang LM, et al. Decreasing clinically significant adverse events using feedback to emergency physicians of telephone follow-up outcomes. Ann Emerg Med 2005;45(1):15–23.

49. Rezvyy G, Parniakov A, Fedulova E, et al. Correcting biases in psychiatric diagnostic practice in Northwest Russia: comparing the impact of a general educational program and a specific diagnostic training program. BMC Med Educ 2008;8:15.

50. Fridriksson S, Hillman J, Landtblom AM, et al. Education of referring doctors about sudden onset headache in subarachnoid hemorrhage. A prospective study. Acta Neurol Scand 2001;103(4):238–42.

The Outpatient Physical Examination

Maja K. Artandi, MD[a], Rosalyn W. Stewart, MD, MS, MBA[b,c,*]

KEYWORDS

- Annual physical examination • Problem-focused physical examination
- Low back pain examination • Dizziness examination • Headache examination
- Shoulder examination

KEY POINTS

- The annual physical examination in the outpatient setting is a valuable tool, despite lack of evidence-based support. It has a therapeutic effect.
- A targeted or problem-oriented physical examination has important diagnostic value, helping to rule in or rule out differential diagnoses.
- Obtaining a careful history is a crucial part of the work-up of any medical complaint and can help narrow the differential diagnosis.
- With a problem-oriented differential diagnosis, physical examination maneuvers can be performed to support or refute a specific diagnosis.

INTRODUCTION

Most of the health care delivery in the United States happens in the outpatient setting.

According to Centers for Disease Control and Prevention data, the number of outpatient visits in 2013 was approximately 920 million, and 53.2% of these visits were made with primary care physicians.[1]

Patients generally make an appointment with their health care provider for an acute problem, a checkup, or management of a chronic condition. It is common that a patient brings a multitude of complaints to a provider's attention. Appointment time is limited, however, averaging approximately 15 minutes per visit.[2] It is crucial that a provider is efficient and addresses the patient's most pressing concerns while conveying a sense of caring. An astute medical provider can gain significant insight about a patient through observation. What is the patient's appearance? Is the patient dressed

Disclosure Statement: The authors report no declaration of interest.
[a] Department of Medicine, Stanford University, 211 Quarry Road, Hoover Pavilion, Suite 301, Palo Alto, CA 94304, USA; [b] Department of Medicine, Johns Hopkins University, 601 North Caroline Street, JHOC 7143, Baltimore, MD 21287, USA; [c] Department of Pediatrics, Johns Hopkins University, 601 North Caroline Street, JHOC 7143, Baltimore, MD 21287, USA
* Corresponding author. 601 North Caroline Street, JHOC 7143, Baltimore, MD 21287.
E-mail address: rstewart@jhmi.edu

Med Clin N Am 102 (2018) 465–473
https://doi.org/10.1016/j.mcna.2017.12.008
0025-7125/18/© 2018 Elsevier Inc. All rights reserved.

neatly or disheveled? Does the patient smell like tobacco? How is the patient's demeanor? Does the patient appear sad or depressed? Can the patient walk without assistance? Being curious and making an effort to understand the patient as a person and not just someone with a disease make a big difference in developing comfort and trust.

This article uses a few of the most common reasons patients present to a primary care physician to demonstrate that the physical examination not only is a crucial tool to help make or narrow down a diagnosis but also it can have a therapeutic effect.[3]

THE ANNUAL PHYSICAL EXAMINATION
Patient Case

A 45-year-old healthy man without any significant family history contacts you, asking if he needs to schedule an annual physical examination. He has not been seen in your office for more than 2 years. What do you tell him?

Beginning in the 1910s, the physical examination has been necessary for work clearance.[4] Since the 1920s, when it was endorsed by the American Medical Association, the general physical examination has been popular with patients and physicians as a means to identify and screen for diseases before they become clinically significant.[5] For the next 50 years, the comprehensive physical examination of apparently healthy people, or the preventive physical examination, was the standard of care. As early as 1975, however, the value of the comprehensive physical examination was called into question.[6] Over the next 10 years, multiple major medical associations, including the Canadian Task Force On The Periodic Health Examination, the American College of Physicians, the American Medical Association, and the US Preventive Services Task Force (USPSTF), released statements recommending against the annual physical examination. Instead, it was recommended to screen for health problems in a more selective fashion.[7–10]

Numerous studies have shown that the annual physical examination does not reduce mortality or morbidity and can lead to unnecessary follow-up studies.[11] A majority of patients and physicians, however, continue to believe in the importance of the annual physical examination. An estimated one-third of US adults receive an annual physical examination, accounting for approximately 8% of all ambulatory visits. This equates to a cost of approximately $7 billion.[12] When patients schedule an appointment for their annual checkup, they expect a complete physical examination and are disappointed when this is not done. Patients' satisfaction with their medical care decreases if the expectation for services has not been fulfilled.[13,14]

What do patients expect during a full physical examination? In a study about public expectations and attitudes,[15] more than 90% of the respondents desired blood pressure measurement, heart and lung examinations, reflex testing, and an abdominal examination. Most of these examination maneuvers, however, are not recommended.[7–10] Systematic reviews of the evidence for the components of the annual physical examination informed the current recommendations.[16–18] Currently, the USPSTF recommends only 4 components of the physical examination[19–23]: measurement of the blood pressure at least every 2 years, Papanicolaou smear for sexually active women with a cervix every 3 years to 5 years up to age 65 years, measurement of weight, and periodic screening for depression. The USPSTF recommends against Papanicolaou smears in women without a cervix or in women older than age 65 years, pelvic examination for the detection of ovarian cancer, testicular examinations for the detection of testicular cancer, thyroid examination for the detection of thyroid cancer, and abdominal palpation for the detection of pancreatic cancer. There is insufficient evidence for skin cancer screening, breast examination when a mammogram is available, mouth examination for oral cancer, eye examination for impaired visual acuity or glaucoma, and hearing examination for hearing loss. Most physicians include many other examination components in their general physical examination that are not recommended. There might be some benefit to checking the pulse in people over age 65 years to screen for atrial fibrillation. Not recommended are palpation of liver and spleen to assess for hepatosplenomegaly, palpation of lymph nodes to screen for malignancy, routine evaluation of reflexes and sensation to assess for peripheral neuropathy, auscultation of the heart for coronary artery disease, abdominal auscultation to evaluate for renovascular hypertension/renal artery stenosis, and assessment of spine mobility to evaluate the risk for low back pain.[16–18]

There are several reasons physicians continue to perform a screening physical examination despite the lack of evidence. Fear of missing a subclinical illness and the notion that most patients expect a head-to-toe examination contribute to the reluctance of omitting the examination. The physical examination is believed a crucial contributor to the patient-physician relationship.[24] Examining a patient communicates a special sense of caring to the patient.[25] The "laying on of hands" while performing a physical examination conveys empathy and solidarity.[26] Commonly, patients express a sense of gratitude and relief when a thorough physical examination has been performed and no abnormalities have been found. Patients frequently state that they feel much better after a complete physical examination. Performing a thorough and gentle physical examination has an important therapeutic effect that should not be underestimated.[3]

PROBLEM-FOCUSED PHYSICAL EXAMINATIONS

The complaint-driven or problem-driven physical examination is a valuable diagnostic tool in the outpatient setting. Many diagnoses can be made by a careful physical examination without diagnostic tests. Examples include cellulitis, shingles, Bell palsy, and Parkinson disease.[27] For many other medical problems, the physical examination guides necessary further work-up (eg, Is a chest radiograph required in a patient with a cough?).

The Problem-Oriented Examination: Dizziness

Patient case
A 48-year-old healthy old woman presents with intermittent dizziness. She denies any recent illness or injury. She takes no medication and has no history of depression. Symptoms are provoked with lying down and looking to the right. She denies imbalance with standing or walking. How do you determine the likely cause of her dizziness?

Although dizziness is a common primary care complaint,[28,29] it is often difficult for patients to describe their symptoms. Determining the timing (onset, duration, and evolution of dizziness) and triggering factors (actions, movements, and situations) that provoke dizziness can help classify the dizziness as peripheral or central.[30,31] It is also important to determine whether there is hearing loss or any additional neurologic symptoms. The history can help narrow the differential diagnosis. For example, disequilibrium (abnormal sense of equilibrium often confused with dizziness) can be caused by decreased visual acuity and signs of peripheral neuropathy. **Table 1** lists a brief differential diagnosis for dizziness as well as physical examination maneuvers that help support specific diagnoses.

Table 1
Dizziness differential diagnosis and physical examination maneuvers

Peripheral causes	
BPPV	Dix-Hallpike[32] maneuver causing transient upbeat-torsional nystagmus. If negative, a supine roll test[33] should be performed.
Vestibular neuritis	Spontaneous horizontal nystagmus or a mixture of spontaneous horizontal nystagmus and rotatory nystagmus is seen. A positive head-thrust test and suppression of the nystagmus with the visual fixation test.[33] Visual fixation can be tested by asking a patient to focus on an object in the room (nystagmus stops) and then placing a blank sheet of paper in front of the patient's face (nystagmus returns).
Meniere disease	Eye examination demonstrates unidirectional, horizontal-torsional nystagmus.[34] There is also hearing loss and balance or gait difficulty.
Central causes	
Vestibular migraine	Spontaneous episodes of vertigo are associated with migraine headaches. The physical examination is normal in patients with vestibular migraine, unless presenting during a vestibular migraine. At that time, there may be a positive Romberg test.
Cerebrovascular disease/ stroke	The use of the HINTS examination can distinguish a stroke (central cause) from peripheral cause.[35] Nystagmus associated with a central lesion, such as acute stroke, is unsuppressed by visual fixation.[33] Skew deviation (vertical eye misalignment, or vertical strabismus) is assessed with the cover/uncover test and is also positive in some strokes.
Cerebellopontine angle and posterior fossa meningiomas	Nystagmus and positive Romberg test without hearing loss
Other causes	
Psychiatric	Normal examination and history of major depression, anxiety disorder, and somatization disorder
Orthostatic hypotension	Blood pressure measured while the patient is standing and supine. Orthostatic hypotension is present when the systolic blood pressure decreases 20 mm Hg, the diastolic blood pressure decreases 10 mm Hg, or the pulse increases 30 beats per minute after going from supine to standing for 1 minute.[36]

The physical examination can distinguish benign from serious causes requiring additional evaluation. Observe a patient's station and gait. When assessing gait, patients with vestibular neuritis tend to veer toward the affected side. An inability to walk, however, is a red flag for a central cause. Orthostatic hypotension can be ruled out by checking the blood pressure with a patient supine and after standing for 5 minutes. Hearing should be evaluated. Hearing is normal in vestibular neuritis. Evaluate for cranial nerve palsies, weakness, reflex changes, ataxia, decreased sensation in the feet, and gait abnormalities. Additional maneuvers can help determine the cause of dizziness. A head thrust is performed while a patient is sitting. During this maneuver, the head is thrust 10° to the right and then to the left while the patient's eyes remain fixed on the examiner's nose. If a saccade occurs, the etiology of the dizziness is likely peripheral.[33] Benign paroxysmal positional vertigo (BPPV) is diagnosed with the Dix-Hallpike maneuver.[32] Transient upbeat-torsional nystagmus during or after the maneuver is diagnostic, especially if the description of the timing and trigger is consistent BPPV. A negative result does not necessarily rule out BPPV if the timing and triggers are consistent with BPPV.[37] In these cases, a supine roll test[33] should be performed.

The head-impulse–nystagmus –test-of-skew (HINTS) examination can help differentiate a peripheral cause of vestibular neuritis from a central cause.[33,35] Spontaneous nystagmus that is dominantly vertical or torsional or that changes direction with the gaze (gaze-evoked bidirectional) suggests a central etiology. With central pathology, nystagmus changes direction less than half of the time[38] and can be suppressed with a fixation test.[39] Test of skew is performed by asking the patient to look straight ahead and then cover and uncover each eye. Vertical deviation of the covered eye after uncovering is abnormal. Although this is not a sensitive test for central pathology, an abnormal result is fairly specific for brainstem involvement.

The Problem-Oriented Examination: Shoulder Pain

Patient case
A 67-year-old woman presents to the clinic with acute on chronic right shoulder pain. The pain got significantly worse after she hung up her curtains a week ago. Now, she has severe pain in the shoulder with moving the arm and feels that the right arm is weaker. How do you evaluate her?

After back and knee pain, shoulder pain is the third most common musculoskeletal reason for primary care visits. The lifetime prevalence for shoulder pain is as high as 70%; 16% percent of all musculoskeletal complaints presenting to the outpatient clinic are shoulder complaints.[40]

The shoulder joint is the most mobile joint in the body. This flexibility makes the shoulder more susceptible to instability and injury. An experienced health care provider can diagnose or narrow the differential of shoulder pain by getting a good history and performing a thorough physical examination. Many clinicians, however, are not comfortable examining the shoulder because the shoulder examination is perceived to be confusing. More than 100 tests have been described to examine the shoulder.

Knowledge of the functional anatomy of the shoulder is crucial to understanding the possible etiologies of shoulder pain. The shoulder joint is comprised of the following structures:

- 3 bony structures: humerus, scapula (with acromion and coracoid process), and clavicle
- 3 main joints: glenohumeral, sternoclavicular, and acromioclavicular (AC)
- 4 rotator cuff muscles: supraspinatus (abduction), infraspinatus (external rotation), teres minor (external rotation, adduction), and subscapularis (adduction, internal rotation)
- The subacromial bursa, which serves as a cushion for the rotator cuff tendons as they move below the acromion)

A good history can give significant clues about the etiology of the shoulder pain.[41,42] Factors that need to be assessed are

Age of the patient: it is rare for patients under the age of 40 to have rotator cuff disease without antecedent trauma.
Location of the pain: pain in the deltoid region is often caused by rotator cuff disease. Pain in the anterior-superior area of the shoulder is frequently associated with AC joint pathology.

Radiation: radiation of pain past the elbow suggests a neurologic problem.

History of activities or trauma

Exacerbating and alleviating factors: for example, pain with overhead reaching and at night is common in patients with rotator cuff disease

The physical examination of the painful shoulder should always include the following steps[43,44]:

Inspection: it is crucial to expose the entire shoulder and always compare to the other side. The shoulder is examined for asymmetry and muscular atrophy. Infraspinatus atrophy can be easily identified by a greater prominence of the scapular spine on the atrophied side.

Palpation: palpation can reveal areas of local tenderness. Isolated pain with palpation over the AC joint suggests AC joint pathology. Tenderness to palpation over the subacromial bursa occurs with rotator cuff pathology.

Range of motion: range-of-motion testing includes flexion, abduction, adduction, external rotation, and internal rotation. It is easiest for an examiner to demonstrate to a patient the movement to be performed and ask the patient to mirror it. If the patient has no problems performing active range of motion, testing passive range of motion is unnecessary. Loss of active range of motion with intact passive range of motion is suggestive of rotator cuff disease. Loss of active and passive range of motion is indicative of adhesive capsulitis.

Provocative and strength tests

Rotator cuff impingement (tendinopathy): inflammation and pain are caused by compression of the rotator cuff tendons (most frequently the supraspinatus tendon) as they cross between the acromion and the humeral head. Impingement signs reproduce the subacromial pain by compressing the tendons between the acromion and the humeral head. The painful arc test (the patient is asked to abduct the arm—pain should be present between 60°–120°) is the only pain provocative test that significantly raises the likelihood of having rotator cuff disease. The Neer sign (1 hand presses down on the shoulder and the other raises the arm on the same side to 90°) and the Hawkins sign (the clinician flexes the arm 90° in the shoulder and the elbow and internally rotates the patient's arm) are the most popular. Neither sign significantly increases the likelihood of rotator cuff tendinitis but the absence of both signs significantly decreases the likelihood.

Rotator cuff tear: besides advanced age (60 years or older) the findings that most significantly increase the probability of rotator cuff tears are a positive dropped arm test and a positive external rotation lag test. The dropped arm test is performed with the clinician passively abducting the arm above 180°. The patient is then asked to actively lower the arm. The test is positive, indicating a supraspinatus tear, when the patient is not able to slowly lower the arm to more than 100°, after which the arm often falls to the side. In the external rotation lag test, the patient is asked to fully externally rotate the arms at their sides. In a positive test, the patient is unable to hold this position because of damage to the infraspinatus muscle.

AC joint pain: the cross-body adduction test increases the probability of AC joint disease. The test is performed with the clinician maximally adducting the affected arm across the patient's chest. The test is positive when the patient has pain in the AC joint.

Table 2 lists the presentation of shoulder pain and associated physical examination maneuvers.

Table 2
Presentation and examination

Cause of Shoulder Pain	Symptom	History	Physical Examination Findings
Adhesive capsulitis	Intense pain, not relieved with rest, shoulder movements worsen the pain	Age: 40–60, diabetes, or thyroid disorder	Limited active and passive range of motion
AC joint disease	Pain at the AC joint		Positive cross-body adduction test
Impingement (rotator cuff tendinopathy)	Lateral deltoid pain Pain worse at night Pain worse with overhead movement History of repetitive activity over the head		Painful arc (Hawkins test, Neer test)
Rotator cuff tear	Weakness Pain at night	Trauma in younger patients Symptoms came on suddenly	Weakness with active range of motion Dropped arm test External rotation lag Internal rotation lag

DISCUSSION

Until recently, the physical examination, next to patient history, was the most important tool a physician had to establish a diagnosis. Recently, the focus has shifted toward technological data. Even in the ambulatory setting, it is frequently much easier for a physician to order a diagnostic test than to perform a thorough physical examination. Reasons for this could be time constraints or that physicians do not trust their physical examination skills as much as they trust the results of a diagnostic test. Lack of confidence in examination skills leads to lack of comfort with performing an examination and to a lower threshold of ordering diagnostic studies.

Despite the impressive advances in clinical investigative technology, however, the physical examination remains a crucial diagnostic tool. In addition to the importance for the patient/physician relationship, a well-performed physical examination can lead to diagnostic clues that would have been missed by just looking at a patient's chart and test results. Developing, maintaining, and teaching strong physical examination skills remain important parts of medicine.

REFERENCES

1. Centers for Disease Control and Prevention. FastStats Homepage. 2016. Available at: https://www.cdc.gov/nchs/fastats/default.htm. Accessed November 4, 2013.
2. Tai-Seale M, McGuire TG, Zhang W. Time allocation in primary care office visits. Health Serv Res 2007;42(5):1871–94.
3. Verghese A, Brady E, Kapur CC, et al. The bedside evaluation: ritual and reason. Ann Intern Med 2011;155(8):550–3.
4. Nugent A. Fit for work: the introduction of physical examinations in industry. Bull Hist Med 1983;57(4):578.
5. Emerson H. Periodic medical examinations of apparently healthy persons. J Am Med Assoc 1923;80(19):1376–81.

6. Frame PS, Carlson SJ. A critical review of periodic health screening using specific screening criteria. Part 1: selected diseases of respiratory, cardiovascular, and central nervous systems. J Fam Pract 1975;2(1):29–36.

7. Spitzer W. Canadian task force on the periodic health examination: final report. Can Med Assoc J 1979;121:9.

8. Periodic health examination: a guide for designing individualized preventive health care in the asymptomatic patients. Medical Practice Committee, American College of Physicians. Ann Intern Med 1981;95(6):729–32.

9. Medical evaluations of healthy persons. Council on Scientific Affairs. JAMA 1983; 249(12):1626–33.

10. Hayward RS, Steinberg EP, Ford DE, et al. Preventive care guidelines: 1991. Ann Intern Med 1991;114(9):758–83.

11. Krogsbøll LT, Jørgensen KJ, Larsen CG, et al. General health checks in adults for reducing morbidity and mortality from disease: Cochrane systematic review and meta-analysis. BMJ 2012;345:e7191.

12. Mehrotra A, Zaslavsky AM, Ayanian JZ. Preventive health examinations and preventive gynecological examinations in the United States. Arch Intern Med 2007; 167(17):1876–83.

13. Brody DS, Miller SM, Lerman CE, et al. The relationship between patients' satisfaction with their physicians and perceptions about interventions they desired and received. Med Care 1989;27(11):1027–35.

14. Romm FJ. Patients' expectations of periodic health examinations. J Fam Pract 1984;19(2):191–5.

15. Oboler SK, Prochazka AV, Gonzales R, et al. Public expectations and attitudes for annual physical examinations and testing. Ann Intern Med 2002;136(9):652–9.

16. Bloomfield HE, Wilt TJ. Evidence brief: role of the annual comprehensive physical examination in the asymptomatic adult. 2011.

17. Oboler SK, LaForce FM. The periodic physical examination in asymptomatic adults. Ann Intern Med 1989;110(3):214–26.

18. Virgini V, Meindl-Fridez C, Battegay E, et al. Check-up examination: recommendations in adults. Swiss Med Wkly 2015;145:w14075.

19. Moyer VA. Screening for and management of obesity in adults: US Preventive Services Task Force recommendation statement. Ann Intern Med 2012;157(5): 373–8.

20. Siu AL. Screening for high blood pressure in adults: US Preventive Services Task Force recommendation statementscreening for high blood pressure in adults. Ann Intern Med 2015;163(10):778–86.

21. Moyer VA. Screening for cervical cancer: US Preventive Services Task Force recommendation statement. Ann Intern Med 2012;156(12):880–91.

22. U.S. Preventive Services Task Force. U.S. Preventive Services Task Force Home Page. 2017. Available at: https://www.uspreventiveservicestaskforce.org/. Accessed January 23, 2016.

23. Siu AL, Bibbins-Domingo K, Grossman DC, et al. Screening for depression in adults: US Preventive Services Task Force recommendation statement. JAMA 2016;315(4):380–7.

24. Goroll AH. Toward trusting therapeutic relationships—in favor of the annual physical. N Engl J Med 2015;373(16):1487–9.

25. Bruhn JG. The doctor's touch: tactile communication in the doctor-patient relationship. South Med J 1978;71(12):1469–73.

26. Ball JW, Dains JE, Flynn JA, et al. Seidel's guide to physical examination. 8th edition. St Louis (MO): Elsevier Health Sciences; 2015.

27. McGee S. Evidence-based physical diagnosis e-book. Philadelphia: Elsevier Health Sciences; 2016.
28. Kroenke K, Mangelsdorff AD. Common symptoms in ambulatory care: incidence, evaluation, therapy, and outcome. Am J Med 1989;86(3):262–6.
29. Woodwell DA. Office visits to internists, 1989. Adv Data 1992;(209):1–11.
30. Muncie HL, Sirmans SM, James E. Dizziness: approach to evaluation and management. Am Fam Physician 2017;95(3):154.
31. Newman-Toker DE. Emergency neuro-otology: diagnosis and management of acute dizziness and vertigo, an issue of neurologic clinics, e-book, vol. 33. Philadelphia: Elsevier Health Sciences; 2015.
32. Dix MR, Hallpike CS. The Pathology, Symptomatology and Diagnosis of Certain Common Disorders of the Vestibular System. Proceedings of the Royal Society of Medicine 1952;45(6):341–54.
33. Wipperman J. Dizziness and vertigo. Prim Care 2014;41(1):115–31.
34. Balkany TA, Gates GA, Goldenberg RA, et al. Committee on hearing and equilibrium guidelines for the diagnosis and evaluation of therapy in Meniere's disease. Otolaryngol Head Neck Surg 1995;113(3):181–5.
35. Kattah JC, Talkad AV, Wang DZ, et al. HINTS to diagnose stroke in the acute vestibular syndrome. Stroke 2009;40(11):3504–10.
36. Consensus statement on the definition of orthostatic hypotension, pure autonomic failure, and multiple system atrophy. The Consensus Committee of the American Autonomic Society and the American Academy of Neurology. Neurology 1996; 46(5):1470.
37. Kim J-S, Zee DS. Benign paroxysmal positional vertigo. N Engl J Med 2014; 370(12):1138–47.
38. Tarnutzer AA, Berkowitz AL, Robinson KA, et al. Does my dizzy patient have a stroke? A systematic review of bedside diagnosis in acute vestibular syndrome. Can Med Assoc J 2011;183(9):E571–92.
39. Lee H, Kim H-A. Nystagmus in SCA territory cerebellar infarction: pattern and a possible mechanism. J Neurol Neurosurg Psychiatr 2013;84(4):446–51.
40. Urwin M, Symmons D, Allison T, et al. Estimating the burden of musculoskeletal disorders in the community: the comparative prevalence of symptoms at different anatomical sites, and the relation to social deprivation. Ann Rheum Dis 1998; 57(11):649–55.
41. BurBanK KM, StevenSon JH, Czarnecki GR, et al. Chronic shoulder pain: part I. Evaluation and diagnosis. Am Fam Physician 2008;77(4):453–60.
42. Greenberg DL. Evaluation and treatment of shoulder pain. Med Clin North Am 2014;98(3):487–504.
43. Armstrong A. Evaluation and management of adult shoulder pain: a focus on rotator cuff disorders, acromioclavicular joint arthritis, and glenohumeral arthritis. Med Clin North Am 2014;98(4):755–75.
44. Hermans J, Luime JJ, Meuffels DE, et al. Does this patient with shoulder pain have rotator cuff disease?: The Rational Clinical Examination systematic review. JAMA 2013;310(8):837–47.

The Electronic Health Record and the Clinical Examination

Helene F. Hedian, MD[a,*], Jeremy A. Greene, MD, PhD[b,c],
Timothy M. Niessen, MD, MPH[d]

KEYWORDS

- Clinical examination • Electronic health record • EHR • Doctor-patient relationship
- Physical examination • History

KEY POINTS

- The adoption of the electronic health record (EHR) has changed the clinical examination: history taking, physical diagnosis, documentation of findings, and doctor-patient communication have each been altered by the EHR.
- There is a paucity of evidence supporting the positive or negative impact of the EHR on patient care; the overall impact of the EHR on the clinical examination cannot be tallied as "good" or "evil".
- The EHR now has a dominant role in clinical care and will be a central factor in clinical work of the future. Conversation needs to be shifted toward defining best practices with current EHRs inside and outside the examination room.

INTRODUCTION

Few technologies in recent memory have aroused as many hopes, fears, and grumbles among health care providers as the electronic health record (EHR). The EHR is not a singular entity but a plurality of technologies, formats, and interfaces, and it is rare to find a stakeholder who has a neutral opinion. Patients, physicians, nurses, administrators, and even medical billers all have something to say, for better or worse, about these new medical media.[1–3]

As more physicians, hospital systems, and policymakers rely on EHRs, it has become harder to pinpoint the central logic for their adoption. Is the EHR an

Disclosure Statement: No disclosures.
[a] Division of General Internal Medicine, Johns Hopkins University School of Medicine, 10753 Falls Road, Suite 325, Lutherville, MD 21093, USA; [b] Department of Medicine, Johns Hopkins University School of Medicine, 1900 East Monument Street, Welch 324, Baltimore, MD 21205, USA; [c] Department of the History of Medicine, Johns Hopkins University School of Medicine, 1900 East Monument Street, Welch 324, Baltimore, MD 21205, USA; [d] Division of General Internal Medicine, Hospitalist Program, Johns Hopkins University School of Medicine, Meyer 8-134-H, 600 North Wolfe Street, Baltimore, MD 21287, USA
* Corresponding author.
E-mail address: hhedian1@jhmi.edu

instrument for physicians to communicate more efficiently about clinical care? Is it an educational tool for patients to learn more about their plan of care? Does its true strength lie in its ability to rapidly check medication orders for adverse interactions? Or does clinical decision support hold the key to increasingly accurate diagnoses? Either way, the EHR has rapidly changed the landscape of medicine. The EHR facilitates improved legibility, author attribution, facile storage, and instant retrieval of notes. It allows concurrent use of the medical record by multiple users, improves security and confidentiality, and facilitates research. The medical record is no longer an illegible, fragmented collection of papers stored in the windowless basement of a hospital or clinic. It is backlit, typewritten, and increasingly available for patients and providers to see. Yet the introduction of the EHR into the examination room has altered the relationship between patient and physician. Inserted into the once binary exchange between two people, computers have created a triangular relationship, as provider and patient increasingly turn away from each other and toward the screen.

To examine how the adoption of the EHR has changed the most fundamental unit of medicine, the clinical examination, the authors performed a Medline search using the MeSH headings, "Electronic Health Records" AND ("Medical History Taking" OR "Physical Examination" OR "Clinical Competence"), which yielded 163 articles. These articles were screened by title and duplicates were excluded, yielding 90 relevant articles. One of the authors then reviewed the title and abstract of each article for relevancy, yielding 49 articles. Each of the remaining articles was then read in full by 1 of the study authors, and 25 of these were judged relevant and are included in this review. Using the snowball method, related articles were identified by citations from this primary pool of articles; 29 additional articles were identified and read in full by 1 of the study authors. Of these, 19 were deemed relevant and included. Additionally, 7 articles which were previously known to study authors, but did not result from the primary search, were added for full review. This yielded a total of 51 articles as the basis for the review.

PATIENT HISTORY

One promise of the EHR, which seems to have been fulfilled, at least from the patient perspective, is the ability of patients to shape the clinical narrative through direct participation. Studies indicate that giving patients direct ability to input information can elicit more accurate clinical information. Through the Family History Initiative—which was introduced by the Surgeon General in 2004—patients can collect and print their family history to make it more available to their providers.[4] Patients in 2 different studies were satisfied with or found a computer-based family health history tool useful.[5]

Patients interact differently with a computer than with a person, and this difference can be especially important when disclosing sensitive information. Some patients have reported a preference for entering their responses directly into a computer rather than disclosing it to a person, because they found comfort in the nonjudgmental quality of computer interfaces.[6] In another study in which patients entered their own social history, it was more common for new information to be added into the sexual history, suggesting that providers may be less likely to collect information that is viewed as taboo or stigmatized.[5]

Provider bias can also influence both the collection and the recording of patient data. In a study of 8 Veterans Affairs medical centers, pain scores as recorded by providers were significantly lower than patient-entered scores in patients with a history of diabetes, posttraumatic stress disorder, or depression and in patients who were not white.[7]

The structure of computer-collected and template-assisted patient histories also presents limitations. Some aspects of the patient history are not conducive to a questionnaire format, and the sheer volume of templated questions that do not pertain to a given patient's needs at specific visit can lead to fatigue.[6] Additional factors, such as medical or computer literacy, can have an impact on the relative ability or willingness of patients to record information in a computer. For example, adolescents in India who were not familiar with computers were less likely to report sexual behaviors when completing questionnaires via audio computer-assisted self-interviews compared with an interactive methodology with an interviewer.[8]

Other potential uses of the EHR for clinical history warrant further exploration. The "chart biopsy"[9] is "the activity of examining a patient's health record to orient oneself to the patient and the care that patient has received in order to inform subsequent conversations about or care of the patient."[9] In a paper-based system, this type of record review involved the logistics of archival research and could take a long time, because components of the record might be stored in various physical locations and not immediately available for rapid retrieval.[9] In 1 study, after receiving a verbal handoff, physicians spent an average of 6 minutes reviewing each patient's EHR, with slightly more time spent reviewing complex cases or new consultations.[10] In an ethnographic study of emergency department to internal medicine handoffs, internal medicine providers saw the chart biopsy as a way to defend against potential biases such as diagnostic momentum.[9]

Yet there is concern that the practice can, in itself, promote diagnostic bias. Some critics have warned against prioritizing the "iPatient"—"a virtual construct of the patient in the computer"—over the real patient.[11–13] By practicing a flipped patient model, in which providers review the electronic chart before interviewing and examining a patient, they may create a bias that causes important physical findings to go unrecognized.[12] Providers may also be missing relevant data during these rapid, targeted reviews. In 1 study of medical student data extraction, fewer than 20% of students identified at least 1 of the 2 critical diagnoses of simulated patients available in an EHR.[14] In addition to omitting important information, chart biopsies may also propagate incorrect information entered on a previous visit.

Providers can detect and respond to nonverbal cues in a way that an EHR cannot.[6] The structured data of the EHR is only a piece of what an astute clinician observes in a clinical encounter. When addressing issues, such as medication affordability, mental health, or substance use, these nonverbal cues can significantly alter the plan of care—and give providers a chance to connect with their patients on a human level.

PHYSICAL EXAMINATION

The impact of the EHR on the performance and documentation of the bedside physical examination is uncertain. Physical examination templates have emerged as a tool to produce more thorough, organized, and understandable examinations. For inexperienced clinicians, these templates may improve the precision and timeliness of their documented findings.[15–17] Templates for specialized physical examinations can also facilitate a more detailed recording of findings.[18,19]

Yet the documentation in an electronic template does not always reflect the examination as it was actually performed. In EHR systems, clinicians are more likely to document their findings after considerable time has elapsed from the actual examination, limiting accurate recall. Moreover, EHRs potentiate the use of templated phrases corresponding to portions of an examination that were not actually performed. Copy-and-paste functions allow prior recorded findings to substitute for a current examination—a practice that can contribute to diagnostic bias and potentially constitute fraudulent documentation. One study found that paper notes were more likely to suffer omissions (41.2% vs 17.6%) whereas electronic notes were more likely to suffer inaccuracies (24% vs 4.4%).[20] In a review of electronic VA records, the physical examination was the most common category of copied events and had a "major potential risk of patient harm, fraud or tort claim exposure."[21]

Still, modern electronic health systems that allow the incorporation of multimedia data may expand the ability to record visual findings of the physical examination. Digital images of dermatologic abnormalities, wounds, or other visual findings can be monitored over time and shared through an EHR. The EHR of the future might integrate unobtrusive wearable monitors that transmit physiologic data that feed adaptive algorithms, prompt intelligent alerting, and improve outcomes.[22] The record could facilitate student mastery of the physical examination by encouraging symptom-oriented and sign-oriented differential diagnosis and suggesting discriminatory examination maneuvers with links to instructional content or exemplar findings. If the pitfalls of copy-and-paste errors and the documentation of findings that were not truly observed can be avoided, the EHR offers significant potential for enhancing physical diagnosis.

CLINICAL DOCUMENTATION

One of the most basic claims of EHRs is to improve clinical encounters through a more functional, accessible, and useful form of documentation, an aspiration that is written into the name, EHR, itself. Yet providers and patients alike have warned that the shift from paper to EHRs generates new problems in the proliferation of documentation of dubious quality.

In contrast to the paper chart, EHRs allow patients to access their own charts with greater ease, thus offering the promise of increasing the scope and granularity of relevant information by including patient-generated data. In 1 study, approximately 20% of patient-generated medical diagnoses and 11% of surgical ones provided a "sufficiently granular piece of data that was deemed to be likely accurate based on chart review by a content expert."[5] Yet much of these useful new data were redundant and could be found—uncoded—in narrative sections of the chart. Importantly, 19% of patient-entered diagnoses were determined to be false. This prompts a complex discussion of how to know if patient data should be trusted if they contradict EHR findings.[5]

Another series of studies characterized the use of EHR templates to drive more effective documentation of history, physical examination, and therapeutic strategies. One study of the use of the EHR in pediatrics found that the inclusion of an EHR-based social history template led to documentation of social history screening in more than 80% of visits, with 30% of the encounters leading to documentation of 1 or more relevant risk factors.[23] Templates may also improve the assessment and plan for certain conditions. For example, an obesity intake protocol and EHR-based weight management strategy was found to be linked with greater clinician weight loss counseling in adults.[24]

A limitation of this study design, however, is that the outcomes depend on documentation in the EHR.[25] Interpretation of such studies requires caution lest the EHR serve as a loop, where documentation is a substitute for behavior and templates that increase documentation are seen as effective. Evidence that EHR templates actually improve clinical outcomes is hard to find. A 2012 systematic review screened 9207 articles and found only 10 that met inclusion criteria. The authors found "very little empirical evidence in support of structuring the history, no evidence of associated risks, and no formal investigations of either benefits or risks from coding the history."[26]

Other studies have documented the risks associated with poor-quality and copy-paste data entry in evaluating the trustworthiness of EHR documentation. In a review of clinical histories on radiology request forms in the EHR of an academic medical center, 18% of clinical histories were cloned, inappropriate, or both.[27] Implementation of an intervention using laminated sticky notes helped reduce the frequency of cloned and inappropriate clinical histories.[28] In another study, providers found e-prescribing systems for tracking formulary, benefit data, and medication lists highly unreliable compared with their prior experience with paper charts.[29]

These negative findings do not mean that electronic media is not useful for clinical documentation, but they point out that both the interface and the quality of data input need to be improved substantially to realize this benefit. Furthermore, attention needs to be given to the competencies and skills required to make optimal use of the EHR. For example, in a physician self-assessment survey, overall computer literacy was most strongly associated with EHR literacy.[30] Several investigators call for new articulations of EHR-based competencies in medical education.[31–33]

DOCTOR-PATIENT RELATIONSHIP

Many clinicians worry about the increasingly dominant role the computer plays in their interactions with patients. The EHR has the tendency to draw a provider's attention away from the patient and to the computer, impairing the ability to meticulously observe subtle signs of disease or discomfort. Doctors spend more time interacting with and inputting data into the computer than they do in direct patient care. Whereas in 1971, interns spent 14.5% of their total working time in direct interactions with patients or relatives,[34] this decreased to 11% in 2000[35] and 9.4% in 2016.[36] By comparison, the amount of time interns spend on charting and forms has risen from 20.5% in 1971[34] to 24% (for chart review and documentation) in 2000.[35] In 1 study, medical interns spent 12% of their time in direct patient care and 40% of their time using the computer.[37] In 1 ambulatory practice, 27% of total office time was spent face to face with patients and 49% was spent with the computer.[38]

Yet the computer is not necessarily seen by patients as an intrusion.[39] In 1 academic pediatric practice, parents of patients whose doctors used an EHR were more frequently encouraged to talk about their worries. There was no difference in parent satisfaction between computer-based and paper-based visits.[40] After introducing the computer at another practice, patients reported a significant increase in overall satisfaction with their PCP compared with baseline. They were also more likely to be satisfied with how medical information was communicated to them and with their comprehension of the diagnosis and treatment plan.[41] Patient perception of the impact of the EHR may be modulated by a physician's level of training. Patients of graduate trainees were more likely than patients of faculty to agree that the computer adversely affected the amount of time their provider spent talking to, looking at, and examining them.[42]

Physicians consistently report a negative effect of the EHR on the patient-physician relationship. In contrast, patients seem either indifferent to its effect or report neutral to positive levels of satisfaction with their care. Through before-and-after qualitative interviews with family medicine residents and faculty, Doyle and colleagues[43] demonstrated that prior to installation, physicians reported concern about the impact of reduced eye contact and about the patients' reaction to their use of the computer. After installation, the investigators wrote, "instead, physicians noted that many of their patients seemed oblivious to the EHR; when patients were aware of it, they appeared to accept and appreciate it." Access to the EHR in an examination room facilitated patient engagement; patients were better able to understand and monitor their health, which led to greater collaboration as patient and provider selected a treatment plan. At 1 large academic health system, one of the physicians' chief concerns before and after EHR implementation was the rapport they established with their patients.

In that same study, patients were surveyed after implementation and they "did not perceive an impact of the EMR on communication or eye contact with the physician. Visits were felt to be more efficient because the doctor was using a computer."[44] A follow-up study by the same investigators demonstrated persistent physician concern about the impact of the EHR on patient-physician rapport. Doctors believed that the EHR had adversely affected patients' satisfaction with quality of care—despite patients reporting the opposite.[45]

There is no evidence that the EHR has affected physicians' ability to empathize with patients. Patients perceive physicians as equally concerned for their emotional and physical well-being, and they believe physicians listen carefully when they work with an EHR compared with baseline.[41] In some cases, they believe that providers are more familiar with them as a person and more familiar with their medical history when they use an EHR.[41]

Electronic communication between friends and family is commonplace. Patients are organizing and mobilizing health information on social media platforms on which health care providers are rated, and creative ideas surrounding health and wellness are shared, cultivated, and accessed.[46–49] Perhaps—instead of perceiving dissatisfied patients—physicians are projecting their own dissatisfaction with the EHR onto their patients.

Arguably, the area where EHR use is most often criticized—the examination room—is the place where it seems to have the least impact. The greatest effects of the EHR are likely outside the clinic or hospital bed. Each patient now has a virtual universe of ever-expanding data, which must be reviewed, processed, acted on, communicated to the patient, and documented about. The EHR acts as a portal between patient and physician, which allows rapid communication of results, electronic prescribing with fewer errors,[50] and a secure messaging system.

The EHR has not changed the patient's side of the patient-doctor relationship. It has, however, undeniably shifted what it means for the doctor to deliver health care. Increasingly, doctors are expected to document, extract data, manage a patient panel, and affect the health of a community or a population. In an era when it is possible to be always connected, doctors are expected to do this not only from within the office but from anywhere, at any time. This may be why physicians' overall professional satisfaction has been linked to their satisfaction with the EHR.[51] Often physicians approve of the EHR in concept, but as Friedberg and colleagues[51] demonstrated "having more EHR functions, such as reminders, alerts, and messaging capabilities (a potential marker of system complexity), was associated with lower professional satisfaction."

The growing complexity and connectivity of the EHR has likely had important effects on physician satisfaction and burnout. Many health providers have complained that EHRs and other forms of digital media only add more expectations to the already high pressures for physicians to be continuously connected. Some element of this complaint can be found more than a century ago, when physicians noted that the then-new medium of the telephone created unrelenting pressures to be connected. Yet the screen brings new concerns; as Dr Paul Hyman eloquently wrote, "So on some days...I hope again for that frozen screen and the possibility that today might be a day without the EHR; a day when the realm of what is possible will shrink; a day where it will be just a few medical instruments, the patient, and me—the whole me."[3]

SUMMARY

The overall impact of the EHR on the clinical examination cannot simply be tallied as "good" or "evil". Patients do not seem as distressed as their doctors by the increasingly central role of the computer in their care. Despite the mobilization of massive capital and human resources into the development and dissemination of the EHR, there is a paucity of evidence supporting a positive or negative impact of the EHR on patient care.

Nevertheless, the EHR will continue to be a central factor in clinical work in the future. Thus, the conversation needs to shift away from the perils and promise of the EHR toward defining best practices with current EHRs inside and outside the examination room. Clinicians need to be intimately involved in the institutional design, implementation, and maintenance of their EHR and the structural environment in which it is deployed. Educators need to learn and promote appropriate etiquette in the technologic era of medicine. Researchers need to define outcomes and methods to study and describe the impact of the EHR on patients, providers, and populations.

REFERENCES

1. Donato A. The soul-less note. Acad Med 2011;86(2):157.
2. Meeker BW. Another perspective on EHRs. Is typing during a patient exam akin to texting while driving? Med Econ 2010;87(9):33.
3. Hyman P. The day the EHR died. Ann Intern Med 2014;160(8):576–7.
4. Zazove P, Plegue MA, Uhlmann WR, et al. Prompting primary care providers about increased patient risk as a result of family history: does it work? J Am Board Fam Med 2015;28(3):334–42.
5. Arsoniadis EG, Tambyraja R, Khairat S, et al. Characterizing patient-generated clinical data and associated implications for electronic health records. Stud Health Technol Inform 2015;216:158–62.
6. Pappas Y, Anandan C, Liu J, et al. Computer-assisted history-taking systems (CAHTS) in health care: benefits, risks and potential for further development. Inform Prim Care 2011;19(3):155–60.
7. Goulet JL, Brandt C, Crystal S, et al. Agreement between electronic medical record-based and self-administered pain numeric rating scale: clinical and research implications. Med Care 2013;51(3):245–50.
8. Jaya, Hindin MJ, Ahmed S. Differences in young people's reports of sexual behaviors according to interview methodology: a randomized trial in India. Am J Public Health 2008;98(1):169–74.
9. Hilligoss B, Zheng K. Chart biopsy: an emerging medical practice enabled by electronic health records and its impacts on emergency department-inpatient admission handoffs. J Am Med Inform Assoc 2013;20(2):260–7.
10. Kendall L, Klasnja P, Iwasaki J, et al. Use of simulated physician handoffs to study cross-cover chart biopsy in the electronic medical record. AMIA Annu Symp Proc 2013;2013:766–75.
11. Verghese A. Culture shock — patient as icon, icon as patient. N Engl J Med 2008; 359(26):2748–51.
12. Chi J, Verghese A. Clinical education and the electronic health record: the flipped patient. JAMA 2014;312(22):2331–2.
13. Rosenthal DI, Verghese A. Meaning and the nature of physicians' work. N Engl J Med 2016;375(19):1813–5.
14. Yudkowsky R, Galanter W, Jackson R. Students overlook information in the electronic health record. Med Educ 2010;44(11):1132–3.
15. Lilholt L, Haubro CD, Moller JM, et al. Developing an acute-physical-examination template for a tegional EHR system aimed at improving inexperienced physician's documentation. Stud Health Technol Inform 2013;192:1129.

16. Katzer R, Barton DJ, Adelman S, et al. Impact of implementing an EMR on physical exam documentation by ambulance personnel. Appl Clin Inform 2012;3(3): 301–8.

17. Lobo SE, Rucker J, Kerr M, et al. A comparison of mental state examination documentation by junior clinicians in electronic health records before and after the introduction of a semi-structured assessment template (OPCRIT+). Int J Med Inform 2015;84(9):675–82.

18. Lowe JR, Raugi GJ, Reiber GE, et al. Does incorporation of a clinical support template in the electronic medical record improve capture of wound care data in a cohort of veterans with diabetic foot ulcers? J Wound Ostomy Continence Nurs 2013;40(2):157–62.

19. Pocuis J, Janci MM, Thompson HJ. Improving diabetic foot examination performance using electronic medical record tools in a specialty clinic. Comput Inform Nurs 2015;33(5):173–6.

20. Yadav S, Kazanji N, K C N, et al. Comparison of accuracy of physical examination findings in initial progress notes between paper charts and a newly implemented electronic health record. J Am Med Inform Assoc 2017;24(1):140–4.

21. Hammond KW, Helbig ST, Benson CC, et al. Are electronic medical records trustworthy? observations on copying, pasting and duplication. AMIA Annu Symp Proc 2003;2003:269–73.

22. Bonnici T, Tarassenko L, Clifton DA, et al. The digital patient. Clin Med (Lond) 2013;13(3):252–7.

23. Beck AF, Klein MD, Kahn RS. Identifying social risk via a clinical social history embedded in the electronic health record. Clin Pediatr (Phila) 2012;51(10):972–7.

24. Steglitz J, Sommers M, Talen MR, et al. Evaluation of an electronic health record-supported obesity management protocol implemented in a community health center: a cautionary note. J Am Med Inform Assoc 2015;22(4):755–63.

25. Shaikh U, Berrong J, Nettiksimmons J, et al. Impact of electronic health record clinical decision support on the management of pediatric obesity. Am J Med Qual 2015;30(1):72–80.

26. Fernando B, Kalra D, Morrison Z, et al. Benefits and risks of structuring and/or coding the presenting patient history in the electronic health record: systematic review. BMJ Qual Saf 2012;21(4):337–46.

27. Shah CC, Linam L, Greenberg SB. Inappropriate and cloned clinical histories on radiology request forms for sick children. Pediatr Radiol 2013;43(10):1267–72.

28. Greenberg SB, Linam L, Shah CC. Follow-up regarding inappropriate and cloned clinical histories on radiology request forms for sick children. Pediatr Radiol 2013; 43(10):1408.

29. Crosson JC, Schueth AJ, Isaacson N, et al. Early adopters of electronic prescribing struggle to make meaningful use of formulary checks and medication history documentation. J Am Board Fam Med 2012;25(1):24–32.

30. Han H, Lopp L. Writing and reading in the electronic health record: an entirely new world. Med Educ Online 2013;18:1–7.

31. Mahon PY, Nickitas DM, Nokes KM. Faculty perceptions of student documentation skills during the transition from paper-based to electronic health records systems. J Nurs Educ 2010;49(11):615–21.

32. Stephens MB, Gimbel RW, Pangaro L. Commentary: the RIME/EMR scheme: an educational approach to clinical documentation in electronic medical records. Acad Med 2011;86(1):11–4.

33. Pageler NM, Friedman CP, Longhurst CA. Refocusing medical education in the EMR era. JAMA 2013;310(21):2249–50.

34. Gillanders W, Heiman M. Time study comparisons of 3 intern programs. J Med Educ 1971;46(2):142–9.
35. Moore SS, Nettleman MD, Beyer S, et al. How residents spend their nights on call. Acad Med 2000;75(10):1021–4.
36. Mamykina L, Vawdrey DK, Hripcsak G. How do residents spend their shift time? A time and motion study with a particular focus on the use of computers. Acad Med 2016;91(6):827–32.
37. Block L, Habicht R, Wu AW, et al. In the wake of the 2003 and 2011 duty hours regulations, how do internal medicine interns spend their time? J Gen Intern Med 2013;28(8):1042–7.
38. Sinsky C, Colligan L, Li L, et al. Allocation of physician time in ambulatory practice: a time and motion study in 4 specialties. Ann Intern Med 2016;165(11): 753–60.
39. Alkureishi M, Lee W, Lyons M, et al. Impact of electronic medical record use on the patient-doctor relationship and communication: a systematic review. J Gen Intern Med 2016;31(5):548–60.
40. Johnson KB, Serwint JR, Fagan LM, et al. Computer-based documentation: Effect on parent and physician satisfaction during a pediatric health maintenance encounter. Arch Pediatr Adolesc Med 2005;159(3):250–4.
41. Hsu J, Huang J, Fung V, et al. Health information technology and physician-patient interactions: impact of computers on communication during outpatient primary care visits. J Am Med Inform Assoc 2005;12(4):474–80.
42. Rouf E, Whittle J, Lu N, et al. Computers in the exam room: differences in physician-patient interaction may be due to physician experience. J Gen Intern Med 2007;22(1):43–8.
43. Doyle RJ, Wang N, Anthony D, et al. Computers in the examination room and the electronic health record: physicians' perceived impact on clinical encounters before and after full installation and implementation. Fam Pract 2012;29(5):601–8.
44. Gadd CS, Penrod LE. Dichotomy between physicians' and patients' attitudes regarding EMR use during outpatient encounters. Proc AMIA Symp 2000;275–9.
45. Gadd CS, Penrod LE. Assessing physician attitudes regarding use of an outpatient EMR: a longitudinal, multi-practice study. Proc AMIA Symp 2001;194–8.
46. De Martino I, D'Apolito R, McLawhorn AS, et al. Social media for patients: benefits and drawbacks. Curr Rev Musculoskelet Med 2017;10(1):141–5.
47. Hawkins CM, DeLaO AJ, Hung C. Social media and the patient experience. J Am Coll Radiol 2016;13(12 Pt B):1615–21.
48. Fisch MJ, Chung AE, Accordino MK. Using technology to improve cancer care: social media, wearables, and electronic health records. Am Soc Clin Oncol Educ Book 2016;35:200–8.
49. Spiegel B. 2015 american journal of gastroenterology lecture: how digital health will transform gastroenterology. Am J Gastroenterol 2016;111(5):624–30.
50. Bates DW, Leape LL, Cullen DJ, et al. Effect of computerized physician order entry and a team intervention on prevention of serious medication errors. JAMA 1998;280(15):1311–6.
51. Friedberg MW, Chen PG, Van Busum KR, et al. Factors affecting physician professional satisfaction and their implications for patient care, health systems, and health policy. Rand Health Q 2014;3(4):1.

Communication and Ethics in the Clinical Examination

Sharon Onguti, MD*, Sherine Mathew, MD, Christine Todd, MD

KEYWORDS

- Communication • Ethics • Physical examination • Clinical examination • Autonomy
- Beneficence

KEY POINTS

- Effective patient-physician relationship is built on trust and sound communication skills.
- Observance and application of ethical principles is integral in this process.
- Recognizing barriers to effective communication and developing skills to address is essential in this process.

INTRODUCTION

At the heart of every effective patient-physician interaction is a relationship that is built on trust. Cultivating sound communication skills coupled with the awareness and application of ethical principles is integral to this process. One of the foremost challenges in competent practice is negotiating situations that arise at the bedside when such issues as patient autonomy, differing world views, honesty, and cost stewardship come into conflict. It is essential for health care providers to consider how to detect and prioritize these issues as they advocate for high-quality and patient-centered care.[1]

The following are different patient scenarios that simulate real-life cases we have encountered in our practice and the approach taken to help build an effective relationship in the setting of competing ethical priorities.[2,3]

CASE 1: THE RESISTANT PATIENT

You are on attending rounds and the team walks into Mary's room, a 32-year-old woman who was admitted for an emergent hematologic condition. She has been at the hospital for 3 weeks. She is finally improving and is tired of getting daily assessments. You are about to start examining her and she sternly says, "I was seen by

Disclosure Statement: No disclosures.
Department of Internal Medicine, SIU Medicine, Southern Illinois University, School of Medicine, 801 North Rutledge, PO Box 19628, Springfield, IL 62794-9628, USA
* Corresponding author.
E-mail address: sharon.onguti@gmail.com

Med Clin N Am 102 (2018) 485–493
https://doi.org/10.1016/j.mcna.2017.12.010
0025-7125/18/© 2018 Elsevier Inc. All rights reserved.

two other physicians earlier and I don't think you need to examine me." She is adamant about this and does not want to be touched.

Competing Priorities

1. Patient autonomy: We respect that this patient has the right to decide who to discuss her care with, and who can perform a physical examination on her. It is easy to empathize with her frustration over a long, complex, and tiring hospital stay.
2. Providing high-quality care: Although data gathered by other members of the health care team are helpful, physicians place the most value on observations made by themselves in person. Although we assume everyone is doing their best, the quality of data varies greatly with the experience and expertise of the examiner.
3. Impact on physician approach: The patient's response may evoke a sense of rejection in the physician, which can lead to a suboptimal physical assessment. This negatively impacts the quality of care provided.
4. Honesty: To be paid for their services to a patient, a practitioner must perform a portion of the history and physical in person.

Approach

It is difficult to ethically override a patient's authority unless they seem to be incapable of making decisions. In this case, the patient is simply frustrated with the routine of being a patient, and her refusal is understandable. A general appeal to be allowed to examine her would be asking her to submit to a hierarchy where her autonomy is less meaningful than the power that places the doctor "in charge" of what happens to her. This appeal could be successful in getting the patient to submit to an examination, but would be detrimental to the physician-patient relationship. Instead, a negotiation with the patient about the parts of the examination the doctor is particularly interested in verifying and why those would be important to her care could result in the patient rethinking their decision and allowing the examination to continue. In negotiating with the patient, it is important to acknowledge their frustration and provide reassurance of unwavering support. This requires a significant time investment; reorganizing the structure of rounds to accommodate this is essential.[4]

CASE 2: THE VERY INVOLVED FAMILY

Lillian is a 75-year-old woman admitted with pneumonia and acute hypoxic respiratory failure. She has two daughters and a son who are always present in her room. They are close to their mother and demand to be involved in every aspect of her care. Attempts at performing the physical examination are met with resistance and a need to justify its importance to her children. The patient is decisional, cooperative, and gives consent to be examined without restriction.

Competing Priorities

1. Appreciating a patient's support system: We want to respect the caring relationship of a patient's family in the same way we have respect for the patient themselves, particularly when their actions seem to be well-intentioned.
2. Patient autonomy: Although understanding that patients often act as part of a family unit, we want them to be enabled to make decisions independent of the unit when necessary, particularly in matters concerning their own well-being.
3. Beneficence: Although acknowledging the role the family plays, it is important to recognize when their involvement contributes to a harmful environment by obstructing the course of care.

Approach

This scenario highlights how a family's genuine care for the patient may create a barrier to quality care. It is important to take the time to explore potential reasons for the family's resistance to the health care process and discuss the significance of performing key aspects of the clinical assessments separately with the family. In addition, given the patient's ability to independently make decisions, it is crucial for the health care provider to be able to advocate for the patient's decisions. In the instance where family resistance persists despite taking the necessary steps to optimize the patient's environment one needs to enlist help from the hospital system in the form of the clinical ethics service or social work. These members of the team are often willing to help facilitate a family meeting where the boundaries of a better relationship are negotiated.[5]

CASE 3: "PAIN MEDICINE–SEEKING BEHAVIOR"

The overnight resident is presenting at morning report. It was a busy night and the last admission was Matthew, a 52-year-old man on hemodialysis who is complaining of abdominal pain. He had been seen multiple times in the emergency department with similar complaints in the past year with no identifiable cause. He was thought to be having pain medication–seeking behavior because he persistently asks for more pain medication. During rounds the patient is noted to be writhing in pain. On careful physical examination, he has an acute abdomen. Surgery is consulted and he is taken for emergent laparotomy, which reveals a gangrenous gallbladder and intra-abdominal abscess.

Competing Priorities

1. Patient autonomy: It is important to take patients at their word.
2. Avoidance of deception: We recognize that manipulative or deceitful behavior is a characteristic of patients with chemical addiction, and seek to avoid enabling addictive behavior.
3. Stewardship of health care costs: We seek to avoid repeating low-yield work-ups for patients with complaints that may be functional in nature.
4. Open mindedness/Nonjudgmental attitude: Patients with addictions or difficult behavior rooted in mental illness can receive poor care if their complaints are not evaluated conscientiously with each presentation.

Approach

When a patient is labeled as having "pain medication–seeking behavior" it introduces a stereotype that often leads to simple dismissal of their symptoms without objective evaluation. It is important to remember that these patients present with genuine pathologies as often as any other. The correct diagnosis and treatment of this patient were a direct result of the objective findings on the physical examination. This was crucial in achieving a positive health outcome in the context of a patient in whom we fear manipulation or deceit because of prior behavior. It is imperative to have a balance between a cautious and an open-minded, objective approach to patients labeled with a stereotype.

CASE 4: THE ANARTHRIC PATIENT

Jack is a 71-year-old man with acute Guillian-Barré syndrome who is now quadriplegic, intubated because of chronic respiratory failure, and anarthric. However, he is cognitively intact and has decision-making capacity. His ability to communicate is limited to blinking.

Competing Priorities

1. Patient autonomy: We recognize that a patient's capability to make their own decisions is not dependent on their ability to vocalize their decisions.
2. Communication barriers: The patient's inability to verbalize results in an underestimation of his ability to communicate his wishes.
3. Psychological barriers: Emotional despair associated with a rapidly progressive quadriplegia that rendered a previously high-functioning, active adult suddenly bed-bound and on a ventilator affects the patient's motivation to participate in the conduct of his examination.
4. Physician's perception: Establishing meaningful connections with the patient in the absence of a two-way verbal dialogue is challenging. The sense of helplessness handling the unnerving "silence" in the context of visible suffering is difficult for the health care team, and may cause them to avoid contact with the patient.

Approach

This case demonstrates the challenges of achieving meaningful patient-physician communication in the setting of a nonverbal patient, and the potential for positive clinical outcomes and rewarding interactions if these challenges are directly addressed. The key is to explore innovative ways to boost the patient's communication. In this case, the family devised an alphabet system that the patient used to describe his symptoms. This offered an opportunity to obtain more accurate and detailed information from the patient's perspective. This also highlights the importance of involving family in the communication process. The impact on the patient experience was invaluable. Another aspect is recognizing the significance of nonverbal indicators, such as eye expressions, and the feedback they provide. On the first few visits, the expression depicted an extremely angry affect. Through the strengthening of communication, he later had an expression of satisfaction and deep gratitude.[6]

CASE 5: CULTURAL RESERVATION

Rose is an elderly widow with no children, but many supportive members of her church visit her daily. She says that they have helped her a great deal since the death of her husband 6 months ago. Rose is hospitalized with new-onset atrial fibrillation and high-grade aortic stenosis. The cardiology service offers her a transcatheter aortic valve replacement and describes significant benefits and significant potential complications (eg, stroke).

Rose is having trouble making a decision. She frets and says "I can't understand why the doctors won't just decide if I should have it or not." Her friends take the team aside and inform them that Rose "will never make a decision." She was accustomed to her husband making decisions for her, and since his death, her friends have found it necessary to act in her best interests, discovering that she does not seem to have the ability to make a decision on her own.

Competing Priorities

1. Patient autonomy: We want to empower the patient to make her own decisions.
2. Substituted decision making: If the patient cannot or will not make decisions, we wish to ensure that she appoints/endorses substitute decision makers.

3. Protection from manipulation: We want patients to make decisions independent of factors stemming from the beliefs of their families, friends, or health care team.

Approach

When we think about patient autonomy, we often envision an isolated patient making decisions solely about themselves. However, people often make decisions as part of a family unit, and it is not unusual for individuals to sacrifice their own wants and needs for the betterment of their family. Culturally, women may be encouraged to put their family's needs before their own and additionally expected to let their spouse or father make decisions for them. Patients who belong to a patriarchal family structure can be unequipped to make decisions about their own health. Although this patient seems to be able to communicate and discuss her medical issue, she is not able/willing to make an independent decision. Thus, we must use substitute decision makers to move forward with her care. It is likely that this patient could have a discussion with her care team about whom she would trust with medical decisions, and that she does have friends willing to step into that role. Appointing one of them as a power of attorney (POA) would be helpful in "making legal" the support system already at work in her life. In a case where a surrogate decision maker is not apparent, physicians must act in the patient's best interest and document the patient's inability to make decisions in the medical record.

CASE 6: PHYSICIAN BARRIERS

Alice is 65; she presents to the emergency department with a dissecting aortic aneurysm. She was critically ill, and unable to make decisions for herself. Her son, who accompanied her to the emergency department, met with the vascular surgeons. In his recollection of the conversation, they told him that the choice was to do nothing and let her die or to do a complicated and long surgery that would ultimately allow her to "walk out of the hospital." He gave consent for surgery.

Although Alice survived her surgery, she had many complications including a spinal infarct with resulting paraplegia, acute kidney injury requiring long-term hemodialysis, and ischemic injury to her feet requiring bilateral amputations. Alice has not left the hospital since her admission 2 months ago. She is delirious, moans in pain, and frequently asks staff to "just let her die." Multiple family meetings with her son to address goals of care are met with resistance. The son is angry, stating the hospital "said she was going to walk out of here and now you are going back on your promise."

No one involved in her case from the vascular surgery team remembers making any such promise. There is no discussion of consent in the medical record, only a signed consent form for emergency vascular surgery. The surgeons have signed off, because she has no current active vascular issues they can remedy.

Competing Priorities

1. Honesty: The health care team wants to carry through on promises made to patients.
2. No undue suffering: We seek to alleviate as much pain and suffering for patients as possible.
3. Substitute decision making: When patients are unable to discuss plans and decisions with us, we seek to have a positive and productive relationship with appointed substitutes.
4. Apology: We seek to disclose and apologize for medical errors.

5. Responsibility: All members of the health care team must participate in building a positive relationship with the patient and family.

Approach

In this case, a surrogate decision maker is available, but does not have a positive relationship with the health care team. To discuss the patient's needs, the relationship with the surrogate must first be mended. In some cases, the reason for mistrust or ill will between families and the medical staff is caused by misunderstandings that are corrected in a face-to-face conversation. Here, the issue seems to be a promise that was made that was not realized. It is important to highlight the devastating effect that promises, which physicians can make without much thought with the intention of being reassuring or persuasive, can have on a desperate family. As in this case, what the family hears and what the physicians recall saying often differ significantly in retrospect.

An apology and explanation from the physician or team that originally participated in the discussion would be best, but in complex cases, it is not always possible to identify who those people might be or to successfully ask them to apologize for an issue in which they do not believe they played a role. As the patient's current doctor, you may need to apologize and explain "on behalf" of the teams that have participated in the patient's care. You may want to discuss this conversation with the risk management team at your institution beforehand to get advice on managing the apology and discussion. An invitation to other teams to be present at a family meeting that you manage could encourage them to be involved in a positive way.

A script for the apology in this case could run along the lines of "When your mother was admitted, you were given the expectation that she would heal and walk out of the hospital. This is not what has happened. We want to acknowledge that and we apologize for it." This apology opens the way for the family to ask questions that lead to open dialogue, a better understanding, discuss prognosis, and the way forward. In the past, physicians were counseled against apologizing for errors and outcomes for fear of legal liability. Recent literature shows that transparency about errors and bad outcomes and apologies are key points in avoiding malpractice litigation.[7]

CASE 7: RACISM

Your encounter with Eileen for the work-up of colitis is going well. At the end of your encounter, she thanks you. "You are the first doctor I have seen who speaks English!" she tells you, with relief. She requests that she not be seen by any "foreign doctors" during her hospital stay. "You know what I mean," she explains.

Competing Priorities

1. Nonjudgement: We recognize that our patients have perspectives and priorities that differ from ours.
2. Patient autonomy: A patient has the right to control who is involved in their health care.
3. Honesty: The patient's request is impossible to fulfill in the complex health care system.

Approach

It is not uncommon to hear a patient express or seek agreement with a sentiment that is offensive to us as providers. These moments are uncomfortable, and it is worth thinking proactively about how you will respond. A patient's social views do not subtract from their right to high-quality health care, but the health care team has a right to work in an environment that does not threaten them.

It is incumbent on us to take care of our patients without regards to their personal views. This requires us to find a way to truly care about people who we might not associate with in our personal lives. The empathy required in this situation requires the practitioner to find sources of alignment or similarity with the patient. Finding an area of agreement with such a patient can be extremely difficult, but this challenge is often the nidus of professional satisfaction and growth.

In regards to this patient's request to see only a certain type of practitioner, education about realistic expectations from the health care system is in order. It is not possible for you to comply with the patient's request given the makeup of the health care team and the lack of control you and the patient has over what kind of care they will need and when. Talking to the patient about this reality and sharing your viewpoint on the value of your colleagues may help the patient anticipate and accept care from a wider variety of people. This discussion also places the consequences of the decision on the patient instead of the practitioner.[8]

CASE 8: AGAINST MEDICAL ADVICE

Jeff is a patient with diabetes and severe gastroparesis. To help with his nutrition and stabilize his blood sugars, a nasal feeding tube has been placed and advanced to his jejunum. Tube feeding is started but the patient has told the nurses he wishes to leave against medical advice (AMA). The tube feedings make him feel bloated and give him abdominal cramps. He plans to remove the tube, leave the hospital and "get better on my own."

Competing Priorities

1. Patient autonomy: We allow patients with decisional capacity to make their own choices, even if we think they are poor ones.
2. Public safety: We should act to restrain patients from leaving the hospital if they represent harm to public safety.
3. Future relationships: We want to act in such a way strengthens and improves the physician-patient relationship.

Approach

When patients threaten to leave AMA, it is important to determine their decisional capacity and whether leaving poses an imminent threat to either themselves or others. In those cases, patients can be "incarcerated" in the health care environment. However, if patients are able to articulate the possible consequences of leaving AMA and do not pose a significant threat by doing so, a more supportive role is encouraged. Paramount in these situations is the preservation of a positive doctor-patient relationship, so that the patient feels empowered to care for themselves in the best way they can and also welcome to return to the hospital/clinic if they change their minds about needing help in the future. This might include writing prescriptions for outpatient medications at the time of departure, a discussion about signs and symptoms for which you would encourage a return to the hospital, and avoiding coercive language (eg, suggesting that the patient's insurance will not pay for their admission, a commonly used lie).[9,10]

CASE 9: SUBSTITUTED DECISION MAKING

Harry is admitted with chronic obstructive pulmonary disease exacerbation. He is delirious, requiring bilevel positive airway pressure, and unable to make his own medical decisions. His advanced directives name his wife as his POA, and are vague about whether or not he would want to be intubated in this situation. His wife is contacted and tells the team that she and Harry are separated and talk infrequently. She states he would likely want aggressive measures but not including intubation. Meanwhile, another woman arrives and identifies herself as Harry's girlfriend. She states that since meeting her, Harry has a new lease on life and she thinks he would be willing to be intubated if his condition deteriorates.

Competing Priorities

1. Substitute decision making: We want to adhere to the decision makers appointed by the patient or delineated by laws, such as Healthcare Surrogate Acts, when patients cannot make their own decisions.
2. Transparency: We recognize that patients make decisions about health care in the context of predictions of future health crises. We understand that at any given time, health and family situations may be substantially different from those imagined when appointing surrogate decision makers.

Approach

Although advanced directives convey a sense of permanence, they are documents that patients can change their minds about and rarely contain explicit instructions about medical care. Therefore, when patients are unable to communicate with their health care team, it is important to obtain and read any documents pertaining to the patient's wishes about care and substitute decision makers. Confirm decisions made on advanced directives with surrogates by discussing the current medical situation and how the patient's decisions apply. There may be circumstances that cause the surrogate to feel the patient would make different decisions than those previously documented. If the surrogate may not be acting in the patient's best interests, advocate for the patient by adhering to their documented wishes and asking for support from colleagues or a clinical ethics service. A different surrogate may need to be appointed.

In this case, it seems that Harry's life circumstances have changed since he appointed his wife as his surrogate decision maker. We cannot be confident that his wife knows how he would respond in his current situation. A discussion with both parties can resolve these conflicts; given their estrangement, Harry's wife might agree to step down as POA and let his girlfriend be the surrogate decision maker. If the conflict cannot be resolved by a discussion with the competing surrogates, the health care team must act in the patient's best interests. In the case of a chronic obstructive pulmonary disease exacerbation, where a terminal condition is not necessarily present, intubation should be initiated if required, in the hopes that the patient would recover and be able to make his own wishes known.

SUMMARY

In this article, we present a series of patients whose care was marked by frequently encountered barriers to effective and meaningful patient-physician communication.[4] These barriers include those extrinsic and intrinsic to the patient and family dynamic. These barriers cannot be simply attributed to a single party in the patient-physician relationship; they arise in the vast backdrop of complicated medical, ethical, and socioeconomic issues within a rapidly evolving health care system prone to rendering patients and physicians dissatisfied by their experience. We demonstrate a guiding approach for the medical team to support and enhance the patient-physician relationship through thoughtful self-reflection that begins with a key question: *What competing priorities are at stake?* This can help elucidate broader principles at play, remove blame from the equation, and unveil a strategy to break a barrier. Ultimately, we remember that patient-physician communication is an art that is human in its very essence: the meeting space of persons, imperfect at times, but always with the potential to transform what lies ahead into something shared and meaningful.

REFERENCES

1. American College of Physicians Ethics Manual. Part I: History of medical ethics, the physician and the patient, the physician's relationship to other physicians, the physician and society. Ad Hoc Committee on Medical Ethics, American College of Physicians. Ann Intern Med 1984;101:129–37.
2. Singer PA, Pellegrino ED, Siegler M. Clinical ethics revisited. BMC Med Ethics 2001;2:1.
3. Riddick FA. The Code of Medical Ethics of the American Medical Association. The Ochsner Journal 2003;5(2):6–10.
4. Stewart MA. Effective physician-patient communication and health outcomes: a review. CMAJ 1995;15(9):1423–33.
5. Arora NK, McHorney CA. Patient preferences for medical decision making: who really wants to participate? Med Care 2000;38(3):335–41.
6. Branch WT Jr. The ethics of caring and medical education. Acad Med 2000;75(2): 127–32.
7. Kachalia A, Kaufman SR, Boothman R, et al. Liability claims and costs before and after implementation of a medical error disclosure program. Ann Intern Med 2010;153:213–21.
8. Kundhal KK, Kundhal PS. MSJAMA. Cultural diversity: an evolving challenge to physician-patient communication. JAMA 2003;289(1):94.
9. Trostle JA. Medical compliance as an ideology. Soc Sci Med 1988;27(12): 1299–308.
10. Berger JT. Discharge against medical advice: ethical considerations and professional obligations. J Hosp Med 2008;3(5):403–8.

Improving Observational Skills to Enhance the Clinical Examination

Stephen W. Russell, MD[a,b],*

KEYWORDS

- Visual thinking strategies • Art in medicine • Art of observation
- Teaching observation skills • Birmingham Museum of Art

KEY POINTS

- Data support that medical student and resident observational skills can be improved using a museum-based curriculum.
- Visual thinking strategies are validated teaching techniques that stimulate learning and encourage evidenced-based decision making in medicine.
- Art in medicine courses are tools to teach core skills, but have limits to their intended teaching targets.
- Understanding the history of art in medicine courses helps to understand their role in modern medical education.

At first blush, the foothills of France seem an unlikely place to trace the origin of the arranged marriage between art and medicine. Situated in a river gorge 7 hours south of Paris, the Pont d'Arc rises above the Ardèche River, a limestone land bridge guarding the entrance to the valley like a cross-armed centurion. The natural structure is a haven for modern tourists, attracting kayakers and canoers, as well as any number of outdoor adventurers seeking stories along the brush-studded banks of the Ardèche. In December 1994, it also attracted the attention of French explorer Jean-Marie Chauvet. As a 42-year-old spelunker, Chauvet recalled, "it was always the unknown that [led] us" into the nearby caves. On that wintery Sunday evening, drawn by warm updrafts from the unexplored depths, Chauvet and his team wriggled 30-feet down to a soft cave floor, then realized, "this was the summit." A French authority on prehistoric art later said, "they hit the jackpot." That day, Chauvet's team discovered scores of prehistoric paintings, entombed for millennia in a network of caves that spanned 5

Disclosure Statement: Nothing to disclose.
[a] Department of Medicine, University of Alabama, Birmingham, BDB 420, 1720 2nd Avenue South, Birmingham, AL 35294-0012, USA; [b] UAB Medicine-Leeds, 1141 Peyton Way, Leeds, AL 35094, USA
* UAB Medicine-Leeds, 1141 Peyton Way, Leeds, AL 35094.
E-mail address: swrussell@uabmc.edu

Med Clin N Am 102 (2018) 495–507
https://doi.org/10.1016/j.mcna.2017.12.011
0025-7125/18/© 2017 Elsevier Inc. All rights reserved.

football fields. Almost immediately, the cave took the name of its discoverer. The governmental caretaker became internationally recognized as the founder of the Chauvet Cave. As word spread, French Culture Ministry officials descended on the site, preserving the relics for scientific study. Within 6 months, the United Nation's cultural agency granted the caves World Heritage Status. The former stonemason who had left formal education behind at age 14, recalled thinking upon seeing the discovery, *We're dreaming*. To the trained artistic eye of a French authority on prehistoric art, the impact was equally astounding. "I realized I was in the presence of the work of a great artist," Jean Clottes, the scientific advisor later said of the discovery. "It was like finding the work of an unknown Leonardo DaVinci."[1]

DaVinci produced his artistic works of genius during the Italian Renaissance, trading tempura for oil paint 6 centuries ago. The prehistoric paintings of Chauvet-Pont-d'Arc Cave used a palette of charcoal and ochre to capture life of the Upper Paleolithic period, some 35,000 years ago. Similar to paintings discovered in Spain's Altamira region and France's Lascaux Caves, which also depict Stone Age animals, the murals of Chauvet Cave completed a trio of subterranean treasures that offered a glimpse into the life of our human ancestors. Upon seeing one set of cave art animals shortly after their discovery, Pablo Picasso told his secretary in 1954, "Primitive sculpture has never been surpassed. Have you noticed the precision of the lines engraved in the caverns?"[2] The precision of the Mediterranean menagerie preserved in the underground galleries depicts bears and bison, oxen and owls. In the Chauvet Cave, a stack of 4 horse heads drawn in charcoal is shaded with natural pigment, as each horse seems to ripple in bas relief along the rocks. Highlighted in red hematite along one wall, reaching across 1500 generations, waves the outline of a human hand.[3]

The discovery of art on the walls of the Chauvet-Pont-d'Arc Cave "may well change our perception, our thinking about the purpose and the use of cave art," the expert, Mr. Clottes, reflected at the time. So important to France were these cave paintings that the Ministry of Culture, Jacques Toubon, made the announcement of the find himself—in Paris. "The discovery is of exceptional value," he said, surrounded by leading archaeologists of the late twentieth century. "It will help us to understand how human symbolism evolved."[4]

Three years later, in 1997, even as the importance of Chauvet-Pont-d'Arc Cave continued to reveal long-held secrets, human symbolism was very much on the mind of Irwin M. Braverman, MD, professor of dermatology at the Yale School of Medicine in New Haven, Connecticut. "It was the week before Thanksgiving—I remember it exactly—and I was running a Grand Rounds at Yale," he told me from his office in New Haven, recalling the story 20 years after the fact (Irwin M. Braverman, MD, 2017, personal phone interview). In this weekly educational conference for residents training in dermatology, "We would have patients brought in, and they were diagnostic cases we had never seen before. The only person who had seen them was the person bringing them in," he said, describing a common case-based learning technique in medical education. During typical Grand Rounds sessions, though, "we can't ask questions, we can only look. After we've had a chance to examine the patients, we all go to the amphitheater and a resident describes the physical findings. I was running this [teaching session] one day," Braverman said, "and the resident was not describing the case well."

The scenario Professor Braverman described unspooled in a format familiar to anyone who has trained under an apprentice–master relationship. Whether in the field of pottery or painting, mechanics or medicine, one learns the principles of a profession by theory but the application of that profession by practice. One such master in the field of medicine was Canadian physician, Sir William Osler, who taught medical students at the turn of the 20th century and wrote about his experiences at The Johns Hopkins Hospital in Baltimore, Maryland. On this topic of experiential learning in medicine, physicians fondly quote Osler's saying, "To study the phenomenon of disease without books is to sail an unchartered sea, while to study books without patients is to not go to sea at all."[5] More succinctly stating those sentiments about the same time, American humorist Mark Twain wrote, "Good judgment is the result of experience and experience the results of bad judgment."

When it came to gaining medical experience—and the good judgment that sprung from that exposure—the dermatology resident in question that late November day in 1997 seemed not only to be ill-prepared to sail that unchartered sea; the resident seemed, in the teacher's eyes, to be unable to trim the sail. "I was frustrated," Braverman told me, "because here I was teaching this, and I thought the residents were not doing the job that they should be doing. Shouldn't there be a way to get them to focus on what is important and not important? To prioritize new information?"

That's when the epiphany struck him.

I bet if I asked them to describe an object that was unfamiliar, they would not know what was important or not important. So, I took them to a museum. If the idea seemed unexpected to his trainees—"they had no idea why I was taking them there"—the seeds of artistic influence had germinated inside Professor Braverman for decades.

"I've always liked to draw—mostly airplanes—and I've probably wasted more paper than anybody else in the world," Braverman told me as a smile seeped into his voice. "And I don't know why, but I just liked to look at things." He also had a knack for looking at opportunities, then translating those observations into action. When as a Massachusetts teenager he realized that his high school did not offer art classes, he helped to influence a group of students to receive instruction in water color painting at the Museum of Fine Arts in Boston. When he attended Harvard, he found himself creating pen-and-ink drawings in science class from what he observed under the microscope, "for accuracy, not for aesthetics." Soon, his interests spilled over into education.

"I took a course by Kline on logic and statistics" while an undergraduate at Harvard, he recalled. "You were assigned a seat alphabetically, and I thought, I wonder if where you sit could improve your score? So we looked." As would be the case time and again in his well-regarded academic career, he used statistics to support his academic hunch. After applying a statistical model to analyze the final grades of his classmates in Professor Kline's class that semester, he determined, "If you sat in the first five rows, or the first two rows of the balcony, your grades were substantially higher than everyone else's. We went to the professor and said, 'That should change.'" Kline heard him out, but the alphabetical seating arrangements remained.

That same smile crept through Dr Braverman's voice as he delivered the punchline. "Thirty years later, those experiments were repeated . . . and found the same thing. I felt vindicated!"[6]

His career took him from a student at the Yale School of Medicine to a Captain in the US Army Medical Corp, where his interest in "visual things" drove increasingly more dermatology cases his way. "Before long, I was seeing more skin cases than anyone else. I suddenly realized that 'visual things' were what I really liked." The accolades that followed that native interest would come. "At the time [the 1950s], I had no idea what the hell was going on" with these new dermatology cases, "and my compatriots did not either. But they cared less." Caring about patients with skin problems, and what conditions those abnormalities represented, led him to write a first-of-its-kind textbook of dermatology based on his own observations and photographs of patients he had personally examined. Two more editions of that groundbreaking book succeeded it, along with 5 dozen research reports, 79 papers or chapters, and the immeasurable goodwill of students and colleagues. By the time his frustrations flourished over a resident's flaccid dermatology descriptions that late November day in 1997, he had earned the right to take his grievances to the museum.

At the time, Linda Friedlaender worked as the Curator for Education at the Yale Center for British Art. "Using original works of art that no one was familiar with leveled the playing field for all," she told me as she recalled the genesis of Yale Center for British Art project collaborating with the doctor–patient encounter course at the medical school (Linda Friedlaender, 2017, personal email correspondence). But at the time, Dr. Braverman did not know he would be working on this project with his friend. "When I decided to bring [the residents] to the museum, I called ahead. I asked if it was okay to have a discussion in the gallery. They said, 'Bring them over.' By happenstance, Linda Friedlaender—whom I already knew—was walking by. She saw me and said, 'I've been thinking about doing something like that.'" Friedlaender, whose husband was an orthopedic surgeon at the medical school, said, "It had occurred to me that teaching visual literacy and slowing down the learning process, which is what we do with all our [museum] audiences, made good sense to do with medical students as well." She soon joined Braverman in his endeavor, selecting paintings with a narrative focus for the residents to observe, paintings that were "full of details to 'read' and describe," and "could be used to offer an interactive learning experience." Braverman remembered the earliest days of his course, saying, "What she added was the description of paintings. She was able to add a few more details that were quickly overlooked." Always with the original intent of this pilot course in mind, he recalled, "based on the nature of dermatology, we could not overlook the minor details."

For those original residents, the course met Braverman's objectives. After they spent time at the museum, "things started to get better at Grand Rounds." But tapping into Friedlaender's independent interest, the 2 educators wondered if they could improve the observation skills of medical students even before they set foot onto a medical ward. Even before they trained their eyes on patients.

By the spring of 1998, Braverman approached the dean of the Yale School of Medicine with his idea to take less experienced medical students to the museum for instruction on observation. "I'm behind it," the dean told the dermatologist, "although I don't think you can do it." Not because they were not allowed to, but because the dean doubted the course's effectiveness. Still, the dean provided "something like five hundred dollars to fund the study" and Braverman was on his way. The new course he designed provided repeated exposure to the museum over the course of the academic year. After several months, members of the media learned about this unique collaboration between medicine and museums. A camera crew came into the gallery to catch the course in action. Braverman recalled the producer of the television show asking, "'How do you know this works?' I said, 'I don't know, but we're going to test this.' The producer said, 'How?' and I said, 'I don't know. But we'll figure it out.'"

Like his high school days without art classes, his assigned seats at Harvard in Professor Kline's class of logic, and the deluge of dermatology cases in the army when no one seemed to know the answer, Irwin Braverman had a history of asking questions that no one else was asking. When the answer eluded those who might know or simply was not there, he had a way of figuring it out. To get the answers this time, he enlisted the help of a children's book illustrator.

Fresh from illustrating and publishing a children's book, first-year Yale medical student Jacqueline Dolev had both experience and interest to bring to Braverman's budding study. "Visual art was an important creative outlet for me growing up. I was an oil painter," she described to me as she recalled her early exposure to Yale's course (Jacqueline Dolev, 2017, personal email correspondence). "I was also very dedicated to science and especially how it related to human processes. When I heard, as a first-year medical student, that Dr. Braverman was taking students to an art gallery to study observational skills, I knew it was important work and that I wanted to be a part of it."

With a team now assembled, Braverman began looking at ways to prove what his medical students did in the museum actually worked to improve their observations skills. "I designed a randomized, controlled study over 2 years to compare our method with traditional lecture and hands-on clinical workshops," Dolev said. "Applying the scientific method was a very important step to legitimize our technique and validate the theory that observational skills could indeed be taught." Friedlaender added, "Gallery exercises were followed by a classroom program of continued observation and reflection." With the incoming class of Yale medical students organized into intervention groups and control groups, the students began learning how to look.

Still, skeptics remained. "When I casually talked to other students, they loved it," Dolev remembered. "They thought it was fun and different to go into an art gallery and be outside of the classroom. But they didn't think it would make a difference in their medical observational skills. They didn't think it would work."[7]

After 2 years and 176 students, the research trio had enough data to analyze. "We showed the students improved their scores," Braverman said. "And the control group did not change at all." By the scientifically accepted standards of clinical research, the results reached statistical significance. The paper Dolev, Friedlaender, and Braverman wrote explained it this way: "Students in the YCBA [Yale Center for British Art] group achieved higher test scores in each of the photographs used in the examination."[8]

Telling the story 20 years later, Professor Braverman's voice remained gleeful. He did not have to wait for others to replicate the data before taking action. He did not have to wait 30 years to be vindicated. This time, a watching world noticed. Dolev authored the report for the team and published the results in the prestigious *Journal of the American Medical Association*, more commonly referred to as *JAMA*. An article in *The New York Times* declared, "Yale's Life-or-Death Course in Art Criticism" allowed students to consider that "in this class, art often imitates death."[9] If the reaction in the medical and popular press was positive, the supporting statistics, and the students' reaction, confirmed Braverman's decision to continue the course. "As soon as we published it in 2001," he said, "[the course] became a requirement," at Yale School of Medicine.

Friedlaender had reservations about continuing the course at first. "Indeed, I was concerned initially about the sustainability of the program. Having data helped a lot," she reflected on what the course has become. "Getting the study published helped even more, but the individual experiences and self-reflections helped us understand how much the program was doing." Dolev agreed that statistics helped to validate the team's intuitive sense that observational skills could be taught. "Randomizing the students and having a placebo group and having the statistics speak to that," she said, "slowly converted people over that time period. But also gave [the project] longevity."

Even with all of the positive publicity Braverman's course had received, the impact this course would have was not on his mind when the article was published. "We didn't know what it would become at the time. Our only aim was to improve observational skills."

My own exposure to museum and medicine courses would come 10 years later as I returned to my Alabama roots. I had left the comfortable corridors of the University of

Cincinnati—first trained as a "Med–Peds" resident then nurtured as junior faculty—to take an academic appointment in clinical medicine at the University of Alabama, Birmingham (UAB). I hoped to fulfill my training by practicing and teaching internal medicine and pediatrics. In that capacity, while working on a lecture for the residents, I began my own journey to the museum.

Where Dr Braverman had discovered a group of dermatology residents lacking a language of description, I ran into issues of a more personal nature. At UAB, the patron saint of the medical school, and most all things relating to internal medicine, is Dr Tinsley Harrison, a giant of a physician with stooped shoulders and thick-rimmed glasses. Although a native Alabamian, he had taught in Texas and Tennessee, and trained in Boston and Baltimore. Indeed, when Tinsley Harrison was just 4 years old, Sir William Osler told his father (whom Osler mentored and described as "his Alabama student") that he needed to train "his boy to be a teacher of medicine."[10] And train him he did. By the time of Tinsley Harrison's death 8 decades later, he had transformed the structure of medicine at UAB, bringing a culture of teaching at the bedside in the presence of patients that persists to this day. He transformed the teaching of internal medicine, too, writing *Harrison's Principles of Internal Medicine*, which categorized diseases by first discussing the approach to the patient. And he had transformed my family, introducing his secretary to his young cardiology fellow, who did not have time to buy a ring before he asked her to marry him. Decades later, their youngest son, newly home from Cincinnati, working as an attending on the eponymous "Tinsley Harrison Wards," had a curious resident ask, "So tell me about the Dr. Tinsley and Dr. Harrison for whom this teaching ward is named." In my mind, it was akin to asking, "Tell me about the President George and President Washington for whom the George Washington Bridge is named."

To respond to the crumbling institutional memory among the residents, I prepared a lecture for the trainees, which I eventually entitled, "The Art of Medicine." I equated Harrison's mastery of medicine with the mastery of observation handed down across the centuries by Renaissance artists. My own undergraduate understanding of art history exposed me to a palette of painters from which to choose. Not surprisingly, I soon encountered Team Braverman's *JAMA* article. As I dug deeper, I found both the foundation and the fruits of Braverman's work.

JAMA published Yale's groundbreaking work 1 week before the Twin Towers fell. Earlier that summer, the journal *Medical Education* had accepted for publication a description of a similar course taking place at the Weill Medical College of Cornell.[11] Using paintings from The Frick Collection in New York, Dr Charles Bardes led 8 students to the museum for 3 sessions of "meticulous observation and description of visual information." As he described in his article introduction, when it comes to diagnosis, physicians "observe, describe, and interpret visual information," but medical education does not "emphasize the actual skill of careful looking; looking is often assumed." Whereas the Yale experience (which his paper referenced from news releases) focused on narrative oil paintings in which the story of the subject was known, the Cornell experience focused on "the study of the human face" as "the face provides the preeminent expression not only of health and disease but of emotion and character." The Cornell and Frick collaborative of science and art emphasized "a broader conception of humanness, one that incorporates both objective and subjective domains," even if the program did not set out to provide scientific rigor to its methods.

By the spring of 2011, as I prepared my lecture on Tinsley Harrison, educational researchers had toiled in the field of art in medicine, providing a harvest of scientific rigor to support the benefits of the Braverman model. Some of the first fruits came at the hands of Dr Nancy C. Elder, now a Professor in the Department of Family Medicine at the University of Cincinnati College of Medicine. "I believe that we must always be evaluating what we do to make sure there is value in the services we provide," she said recently when asked about her early involvement in evaluating the effectiveness of art and medicine courses, "whether it is the care we give our patients or the education we give our learners" (Nancy Elder, 2017, personal email correspondence). I had joined a long list of residents rotating through her family medicine clinic during my own training, back when her educational responsibilities took her from the clinics to the classroom, and ultimately to the museum. Like most educators, enjoying the love of learning—and teaching—proceeded the search for statistics. "We really started our course out of self-interest," she said. "We believed then, and I still believe now, that observation and description have become lost arts." Like Braverman and Friedlaender before her, "our goal was to slow back down" the process of observation, and in so doing, "to develop skills in cognitive decision making and to practice using it when it didn't matter, so they could hopefully call on that skill when they did."

The resulting collaboration with the Cincinnati Art Museum provided not just a glimpse of statistical significance, but a sense that courses of this nature had staying power. As her team wrote in the introduction to the publication of their work, "the primary goal of the course is to improve communication and observation skills used in the patient-doctor relationship by guided instruction in observation . . . of the visual arts."[12] Using an online evaluation asking graduates of their "Art of Observation" course to reflect on their experience, her study evaluated the course's influence on careers. The survey among 19 students showed that the course "positively influenced clinical skills . . . and led to a sense of personal development as a physician."

Larger statistical fruits followed.

Dr Joel Katz, of Harvard Medical School, published the results of training medical students in a similar course in Boston, entitled, "Training the Eye: Improving the Art of Physical Diagnosis." When his team compared the 24 participating students with 34 classmates not trained to observe in a museum, the results helped to established a pattern, supported by statistics, with courses of this type. Harvard's students not only increased their observation abilities, but also demonstrated "a doses response . . . for those who attended eight or more sessions compared to participants who attended seven or fewer sessions."[13] Once learners crossed the threshold of the museum galleries, teaching them a structure to describe an unknown improved their observational skills. Asking them to reflect on their experience had lasting impact. And repeating that process had more benefit than isolated exposures.

With the tailwind of a successful lecture behind me, and buoyed by the Birmingham Museum of Art looking to collaborate with the medical school on a similar project, I secured a spot from the dean in the medical school's fall lineup of "Special Topics Courses" entitled, "Art in Medicine: Learning to Think by Looking at Art." It had been 10 years since the Yale group sowed the seeds of art in medicine by publishing the September 2001 *JAMA* article, and a decade of medical students had reaped the benefits. Now, it was UAB's turn. In the excessive hubris that often follows in the wake of a junior faulty appointment, I emailed Dr Braverman to share the good news. In the accessible humility that sets apart senior faculty of great respect, he responded within 2 hours. "Dear Dr. Russell, I am pleased to help" (Irwin M. Braverman, 2011, personal email correspondence).

And help he did.

He emailed the original pretest and posttest images, along with the rubric used to grade the students. He offered insights into what had worked well at Yale over the years . . . and what had not. When a member of the UAB team from the Birmingham Museum of Art met him at a conference, he shared with her his view that training students early in their education—as first-year students and not Thanksgiving-era residents—could have more of an impact before bad observational habits set in.

Combining what we considered the best of the published articles in the medicine curricula, and with the expressed objective "To improve the observational skills of medical students by studying visual arts," we offered a variety of visual experiences to teach the lessons. Like other courses before us, students learned to look in lectures and then applied their skills in the galleries. Because most of our students had completed 2 years of basic science training and had had a taste of clinical medicine, we made explicit the connection of medicine and art. On Day One, we stepped back 6 centuries, decades before DaVinci's birth, to make a diagnosis from an altarpiece.

In the history of Western art, few Flemish painters could recreate the world they saw like Jan van Eyck. With his emphasis on accurate observations from the natural world, van Eyck pivoted the art world from idealism and iconography to the dawn of realism in the Renaissance. Patrons did not shy away from his forthright, if at times unflattering, representations. In his 15th century altarpiece *The Virgin and Child with Canon van der Paele* (**Fig. 1**), van Eyck paints his aged patron amid the saints in what would come to be the last years of the clergyman's life. As the UAB students study images of the painting, they are asked to simply write down what physical examination abnormalities they observe, quickly noting the prominent temporal arteries, lateral eyebrow thinning, and soft tissue swelling that van Eyck so precisely painted. Contemporary church records report the infirm Canon van der Paele being unable to perform his morning duties. As our collective list of physical examination abnormalities grew, we referenced Hutchinson's 19th century original case report of temporal arteritis, in which "an old man named Rumbold . . . tall, fine looking, rather thin and quite bald" was "upwards of eighty" and had "red 'streaks on his head' which were painful and prevented his wearing his hat."[14]

Two question are then posed to the students: First, based on what is observed, do you think that Canon van der Paele had the same condition that Hutchinson described 500 years later? Second, what evidence, based on your observation, supports that conclusion? At this stage of their training, many of the clinically experienced medical students asked for more. What would the laboratory results have been? The

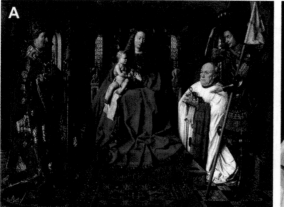
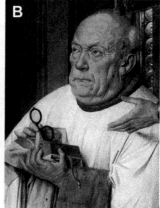

Fig. 1. (*A*) The Virgin and Child with Canon van der Paele by Jan van Eyck. (*B*) Inset of the clergyman from the same painting. (Available via Wikipedia: https://en.wikipedia.org/wiki/Virgin_and_Child_with_Canon_van_der_Paele. Accessed August 1, 2017.)

radiographs? The response to therapy? Of course, the conversation is counterfactual. Preparing them for the gallery, they are reminded that if a man with a paint brush and a gift for observation can stimulate such questions across the centuries, how much more can their own eyes learn from patients simply by taking time to observe.

In learning to look, our next stop is in front of a portrait.

If Flemish painter Jan van Eyck embodied the birth of a new movement in realism, then few portrait artists captured the American spirit at the dawn of the 20th century like John Singer Sargent. Born in Rome to a Philadelphia physician, Sargent discovered his artistic skill as a boy in Florence, and then perfected painting as a young man in Paris. Even though only in his 20s, "word spread that he made sitting for portrait highly pleasurable and affluent women in increasing numbers wish to do so," leading to stunning, if at times scandalous, renderings of his subjects.[15] One of those portraits, painted when he was in his mid-40s, is now on display at the Birmingham Museum of Art (**Fig. 2**). UAB's "Art in Medicine" students gather before the full-length painting to discuss what they see. Standing against a balcony draped with thick fabric, the subject (whose name is initially hidden from the students) stares dispassionately from the portrait. Comments that begin about the subject's garments and postures soon veer into speculation about her social status. The docents facilitating the session steer the conversation with simple prompts, asking students to support their conclusions with

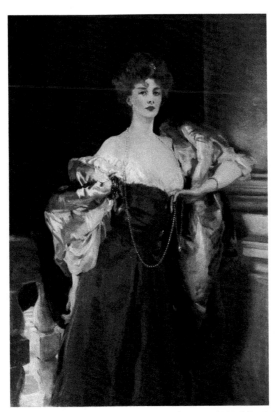

Fig. 2. Portrait of Lady Helen Vincent, Viscountess D'Abernon (1904) by John Singer Sargent. (Available via Wikipedia: https://en.wikipedia.org/wiki/Helen_Vincent,_Viscountess_D%27Abernon. Accessed August 1, 2017.)

what they see in the painting before them. Although many students correctly conclude that Sargent's subject was a wealthy woman of privilege when he painted her in Venice in 1904, they tend to be surprised to learn that Lady Helen Vincent, the Viscountess D'Abernon, went on to serve as a nurse anesthetist in the first World War, reportedly treating thousands of patients during her tenure. Concluding the session, the docents and faculty remind the students that although observation is a critical component of the physical examination, it can often be an incomplete measure of social history.

A third example used to teach UAB's "Art in Medicine" observation uses narrative art from the American Revolution. In 1772, during a time of growing tensions between the 13 colonies and the British Crown, American painter Benjamin West enjoyed the good graces of King George III. Living in London, the Philadelphian had already established his reputation on both sides of the Atlantic, painting portraits of Benjamin Franklin as well as the royal family. In the same year, King George appointed him historical painter to the court, Benjamin West completed a 4×6-foot oil-on-canvas painting entitled *Erasistratus the Physician Discovers the Love of Antiochus for Stratonice* (**Fig. 3**). Recounting the legend of the eminent Greek physician who diagnosed unrequited love in the Prince of Syria, West's painting occupies a place of prominence in the American Gallery at the Birmingham Museum of Art. Without knowing the title, the students use the same techniques of visual observation to recreate a narrative. Using supporting visual evidence, they collectively summarize the painting, typically with a high degree of accuracy. They then learn the title and the backstory of both painting and painter. Making a final effort to connect the galleries to the clinic, students are asked, "Is such a scenario medically possible?" In most cases, the conversation turns to Takotsubo cardiomyopathy, the stress-induced "broken heart syndrome."

Each of the exercises in UAB's "Art in Medicine" course builds on the foundations established by Dr Braverman and his colleagues at Yale, using an educational technique known as Visual Thinking Strategies (VTS). Developed by Harvard psychologist Abigail Housen's decades of research into how viewers consider art, VTS helps

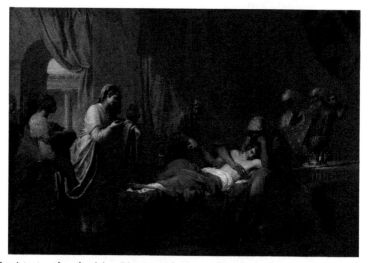

Fig. 3. Erasistratus the physician Discovers the love of Antiochus for Stratonice by Benjamin West. (Available via Wikipedia: https://commons.wikimedia.org/wiki/File:Erasistratus_the_Physician_Discovers_the_Love_of_Antiochus_for_Stratonice_-_Benjamin_West_-_Google_Cultural_Institute.jpg. Accessed August 1, 2017.)

students to learn how to look. By "building from what they [students] already know" in an "active process of trying things out and discovering new ways to construct and build meaning," VTS also propose a structure to aid that learning.[16] The best learning of this type is first-hand experience; students work in groups to consider the works of art. Although teachers want to direct the students' attention, the questions are open ended. And although the museum docents aim to corral the conversation, they want to restate observations from the learners, not interpret those comments. Indeed, teachers trained to facilitate a VTS curriculum ask 3 basic, if somewhat circular, questions about the work being considered: What is going on? What do you see that supports that conclusion? What else is seen?[17]

The UAB experience in front of West's *Erasistratus the Physician* echoes the VTS of courses that came before ours: paintings are chosen for the known history they provide, and students are led down a path of mutual discovery toward a definite conclusion, encouraged to support their theories along the way. Although we cannot know the results of *Antiochus'* echocardiogram—and the look in many students' eyes tell me they still pine for that information—we can know West's original intent from 1772. Teaching the students the value of informed observation, even if it leads to additional investigation, furthers the goal of the curriculum of VTS.

At the end of the day, when the clinics have closed and the gallery lights dim, the educational question remains: do "Art in Medicine" courses reach their objective to improve observational skills? A dispassionate view of the data offers a mixed assessment, depending on the question that is asked. If one asks, "Can medical students improve their observational skills by using a museum-based curriculum based on visual thinking strategies?", the answer is yes. Dolev emphasized the Yale course, and those that followed, is simply "using art as a tool to teach a core skill." Trying to read more into courses of this type can sometimes be problematic.

"I think educational research is still far behind clinical research," Dr Nancy Elder from the University of Cincinnati reflected. "All education exists to change our learners in some way, either short term or long term." Her own 2006 study saw a qualitative impact on the long-term benefit of having taken a course on the "Art of Observation." (She parenthetically told me that the University of Cincinnati was "politely but legally asked to stop using that name for our course" owing to the course title "Art of Observation" being copyrighted by another university.) Braverman wryly commented, "I also feel that Jackie [Dolev] and I are job creators. I know of two people who are actually probably making some money with this technique." His humor came though as he said, "I think that we should be given credit by the federal government. We have improved the economy."[7]

Seven years after Dr Elder published her data, investigators at Chicago's Rush University trained a statistical eye in evaluating a visual arts-based curriculum with their medical students, documenting qualitative improvement of written responses without being able to demonstrate specific improvement on observational test scores.[18] Even among seasoned Art in Medicine educators, surprising trends emerged. Students seemed to be learning more than just observational skills; they seemed to be learning how to think like doctors.

Dr Braverman had run the course at Yale for well over a decade when his team decided to change the questions on the end-of-course survey. The students were asked 2 additional questions: What did you learn about yourself as an observer? And what principles of observation did you learn from this course? "We suddenly realized we were teaching them how to make medical decisions," Braverman told me. "That just blew our minds." Overwhelmingly, students reported that, before the course, they tended to jump to conclusions when faced with a new problem, such as a narrative painting. To counteract that tendency, they learned they had to review information multiple times to get enough information to draw appropriate conclusions. "We had no idea that the real benefit was that they were understanding how to make medical decisions."

That fateful day in December 1994, when Jean-Marie Chauvet and his team unearthed the earliest known record of human art, almost did not happen. In truth, he wanted to turned back. "It was already dark, the air was even colder than in the early afternoon, and we did not feel strong enough," he wrote in his memoir.[19] "So we decided to go home."

But he hesitated.

Motivated by fascination but moored by fatigue, one emotion split the difference: fear.

"The fear of someone else having the 'première' before us" led him onward. He knew he was on the brink of discovery, and he wanted to find out—before someone else did. "We arrived at the edge of the shaft, unrolled our ladder and, one after the other, climbed down into the profound darkness of the cave." It would not be an easy decent. "We moved in single file through the darkness . . . darkness dominated all around us . . . advancing slowly, we redoubled our precautions."

Then, in the light of the headlamp of Chauvet's fellow explorer, "We immediately spotted the drawing of a little red mammoth on a rocky spur hanging down from the ceiling. We were overwhelmed. . . . Prehistoric people had been here before us." The emotions of the moment—from fatigue to fear and now fascination—made them "incapable of uttering a single word. Alone in the vastness, lit by the feeble beam of our lamps, we were seized by a strange feeling. Everything was so beautiful, so fresh, almost too much."

For a medical student examining a patient for the first time in a clinical setting, or a dermatology resident describing unknown skin findings in Grand Rounds, being overwhelmed can seem like familiar territory. Like a late evening spelunker, those trainees can find themselves moored by uncertainty, cultural differences, or simply fatigue. Courses pairing museums and medical students can provide a way forward, a dictionary to describe what is unfamiliar to make it more accessible. If those courses are successful in the service of improving observation, they may even provide more meaning to a budding career.

"Deeply impressed," Jean-Marie Chauvet wrote of that first day of discovery in caves of southern France, "we were weighed down by the feeling that we were not alone." For students learning the Art of Observation—and those who teach them—highlighting that sense of connectedness is perhaps the most valuable lesson of all.

REFERENCES

1. Scott K. Spelunker's passion pays off: Jean-Marie Chauvet and his small team of cave diggers 'hit the jackpot,' finding a cache of Stone-Age art. Los Angels Times 1995. Available at: http://articles.latimes.com/1995-02-14/news/wr-31937_1_chauvet-cave. Accessed July 19, 2017.
2. Bahn P. A lot of bull? Pablo Picasso and ice age cave art. Antropologia-Arkeologia 2005;57:217–23.
3. Thurman J. First impressions: what does the world's oldest art say about us. The New Yorker 2008.
4. Simons M. Prehistoric art treasure is found in French cave. The New York Times 1995. Available at: http://www.nytimes.com/1995/01/19/world/prehistoric-art-treasure-is-found-in-french-cave.html?pagewanted=all. Accessed July 19, 2017.

5. Osler W. Books and men. The Boston Medical and Surgical Journal. 1901.
6. Benedict ME, Hoag J. Seating location in large lectures: are seating preferences or location related to course performance? J Econ Educ 2004;35(3):215–31.
7. Braverman I, Dolev J. "Doctor, doctor: conversations about medicine." Audio blog post. The Art of Noticing. Yale Netcasts; 2016. Available at: https://itunes.apple.com/us/podcast/doctor-doctor-conversations-about-medicine/id1082433585?mt=2. Accessed August 5–6, 2017.
8. Dolev JC, Friedlaender LK, Braverman IM. Use of fine arts to enhance visual diagnostic skills. JAMA 2001;286(9):1020–1.
9. DiGrazia C. Yale's life-or-death course in art criticism. The New York Times 2002.
10. Pittman JA. Tinsley Harrison: teacher of medicine. Montgomery (AL): New South Books; 2015. Print.
11. Bardes CL, Gillers D, Herman AE. Learning to look: developing clinical observational skills at an art museum. Med Education 2001;35:1157–61.
12. Elder NC, Tobias B, Lucero-Criswell A, et al. The art of observation: impact of a family medicine and art museum partnership on student education. Fam Med 2006;38(6):393–8.
13. Naghshineh S, Hafler JP, Miller AR, et al. Formal art observation training improves medical students' visual diagnostic skills. J Gen Intern Med 2008;23(7):991–7.
14. Hutchinson J. Diseases of the arteries. Arch Surg 1889;1:323–9.
15. McCullough D. The greater journey: Americans in Paris. New York: Simon & Schuster; 2011. Print.
16. Housen A. Visual thinking strategies. Eye of the beholder: research, theory, and practice. Paper presented at: Aesthetic and Art Education: A Transdisciplinary Approach. Lisbon, Portugal, September 27–29, 1999.
17. Katz J, Khoshbin S. Can visual arts training improve physician performance? Trans Am Clin Climatol Assoc 2014;125:331–41.
18. Jasani S, Saks N. Utilizing visual arts to enhance the clinical observation skills of medical students. Med Teach 2013;35(7):1327–31.
19. Chauvet JM, Deschamps EB, Hikkaire C. Dawn of art: the Chauvet Cave, the oldest known paintings in the world. New York: Harry N. Abrams, Inc. Publishers; 1996. Print.

Patient-Centered Bedside Rounds and the Clinical Examination

Peter R. Lichstein, MD*, Hal H. Atkinson, MD

KEYWORDS

- Bedside rounds • Relationship-centered communication • Physical examination
- Interprofessional • Patient centered • Medical education

KEY POINTS

- Patients and families prefer bedside case presentations and care discussions.
- Bedside rounds are venues to integrate relationship-centered communication and physical diagnosis skills into the work flow of clinical care.
- Efficient bedside rounds require team and patient preparation.
- Patient and provider experience can improve with bedside rounding.

VIGNETTE 1: THE TEACHING SERVICE

Dr Julie Wells is a newly appointed faculty member at an academic medical center who is preparing for her first block as an inpatient attending. She would like to round at the bedside, but her new hospital has a tradition of conference room or hallway rounds. Dr Wells is wondering how she can convince her new team to give bedside rounding a try.

VIGNETTE 2: THE NONTEACHING SERVICE

Dr George Johnson is a hospitalist at a community hospital. He greatly values the contributions of interprofessional team members in augmenting his evaluation of patients. However, he almost always rounds separately from other providers. Dr Johnson wishes the hospital culture provided more support for interprofessional bedside rounds. He thinks this practice would benefit the team, improve safety, and enhance the patient experience.

Both Drs Wells and Johnson are motivated to conduct bedside rounds with their clinical teams to connect effectively with patients, integrate valuable aspects of the

Department of Internal Medicine, Section on General Internal Medicine and Section on Gerontology and Geriatric Medicine, Wake Forest School of Medicine, Medical Center Boulevard, Winston Salem, NC 27157, USA
* Corresponding author.
E-mail address: plichste@wakehealth.edu

Med Clin N Am 102 (2018) 509–519
https://doi.org/10.1016/j.mcna.2017.12.012
0025-7125/18/© 2018 Elsevier Inc. All rights reserved.

clinical examination into the daily workflow, and make the experience beneficial for patients and their loved ones. They want rounds to be both "patient proximate" (at the bedside) and truly "patient centered" (inviting patient participation; Eric Warm, personal communication, 2017.) This article reviews practical considerations and suggestions to conduct efficient, high-yield bedside rounds. Many of the approaches were developed at Wake Forest Baptist Health with funding from the Josiah Macy Jr. Foundation and the Institute on Medicine as a Profession. The strategies for relationship-centered communication grew out of collaboration with the Academy on Communication in Healthcare.

THE DECREASE IN BEDSIDE ROUNDING

Over the past 50 years, bedside rounding has all but disappeared from the wards of teaching and nonteaching services.[1,2] Changes in medical systems, workflow, hospital culture, and values make Osler's admonition that there be, "No teaching without a patient for a text, and the best teaching is that taught by the patient himself," seem like a relic from a prior era.[3] In many academic medical centers, bedside rounds have been replaced by presentations of newly admitted patients in a conference room or hallway followed by a brief visit to the bedside to meet the patient and confirm key findings. Care discussions of follow-up patients are relegated to "card flip" without the team laying eyes or hands on their patients. Time at the bedside is estimated to account for 8% to 19% of total rounding time.[4,5] On nonteaching services, the situation is similar. Providers round separately on their patients, rather than as a team, and care discussions occur in the hallway or conference room rather than at the bedside. As a result, it often seems that attention devoted to the "iPatient" housed in the electronic medical record takes precedence over care of the actual sick person in the bed.[6]

Many factors contribute to the trend away from the bedside. When care discussions focus primarily on reviewing and interpreting laboratory and imaging studies, teams understandably prefer the relative comfort, privacy, and computer access provided in a conference room.[7,8] In medical systems where efficiency rules, providers may eschew bedside rounding if they think they take more time than hallway or conference room rounds.[9] Work compression owing to duty-hour restrictions for house staff and hospital mandates for early discharges and decreased durations of stay mean that all providers have less time to talk with and listen to patients and families. One study estimates that interns, on average, spend only 7 minutes per day with each of their patients.[10] The bulk of their day is spent in front of computers rather than with patients.

Patient expectations and preferences are rarely a barrier to bedside rounding.[11] Teams are often worried that patients will be overwhelmed by bedside discussions of complex medical issues or upset when sensitive topics, such as substance abuse or pain management, are mentioned in the presence of a large rounding team. Providers may feel uncomfortable about how to manage strong patient emotions, such as anger or grief, and are apprehensive that rounds will be derailed by prolonged discussions of psychosocial issues.[12] Beginning learners are often anxious about making mistakes during bedside presentations.[12] Finally, a generation of clinicians with few or no role models from their own training lack confidence in their own bedside teaching and communication skills.[13]

RETURNING TO THE BEDSIDE

The renewed interest in bedside rounding is evidence based. It reflects the re-envisioning of clinical care that is taking place in many health systems and practices.

PATIENTS AND FAMILIES

Contrary to concerns raised by providers, patients and families overwhelmingly prefer bedside rounds as long as they are conducted tactfully and sympathetically with reasonable attention to privacy and limited use of medical jargon.[12,14] Patients value time with their providers, and bedside rounds achieve this by transposing discussions from the hallway to the patient's room, where they are literally the center of the team's attention. During bedside presentations, patients are privy to and can contribute to the presentation of their case. By conducting care discussions at the bedside rather than in the hallway, patient understanding is enhanced. Seeing that their team is "on the same page" builds confidence and trust.[15] Most patients are willing participants in bedside teaching and actually enjoy contributing to the education of tomorrow's professionals.

HEALTH SYSTEMS AND TEAMS

Health systems that recognize how bedside rounds can enhance patient experience and facilitate interprofessional teamwork are more likely to promote this model of care. Institutional buy-in is needed to facilitate the systems and infrastructure changes that make bedside rounding possible. For instance, regionalization of patients for each rounding team is essential for efficient rounding and can only be achieved with strong support from hospital leaders.[16] Similar support is needed to overcome workflow and scheduling barriers that make it difficult for interprofessional teams to round together at the bedside.[16]

EFFICIENCY

Bedside rounding can be time neutral or even more efficient than other rounding models.[17] Regionalization of patients to one geographic ward saves time wasted in transit. Time is also saved by not repeating at the bedside aspects of the history that have already been presented in the hallway or conference room.[16] At our hospital, attendings on teaching and nonteaching services overwhelmingly view bedside rounding as more efficient and accurate than other models. Time is saved because they seldom need to return to the ward after rounds to confirm findings or hear the patient's perspective; these tasks were already accomplished during rounds. The fear that addressing psychosocial issues will make rounds interminable is not supported by evidence; encounters are more efficient when internists and surgeons convey empathy during office appointments.[18,19] Other time-saving strategies include entering orders before leaving the room and adhering to realistic time limits for presentations (approximately 5 minutes) and total time in the room (approximately 15 minutes). Efficiency is also enhanced when attendings choose to review admission and progress notes before rounds rather than visiting new patients as "unknowns."[16] The attending physician must be mindful to avoid the cognitive biases of premature closure or anchoring on a diagnosis that could occur with this approach. Advance review provides an opportunity for the teaching physician to guide the team in correcting any inaccuracies in documentation after the history and examination findings are probed and confirmed at the bedside. A bedside synopsis rather than a complete presentation leaves more time for teaching the clinical examination and for engaging patients and families in decision making.[20,21]

EDUCATION

The literature is replete with articles extolling the advantages of bedside teaching. Grounded in the realities of clinical care, the bedside provides a uniquely engaging venue to demonstrate, observe, and assess communication and physical examination skills, professionalism, and empathic approaches to patient suffering.[20–24]

JOY IN PRACTICE

Providers and learners frequently report that bedside rounding reconnects them with the joy and satisfaction of practicing medicine. Relationship-centered communication makes the work more enjoyable, fulfilling, and can reduce burnout.[25] Reinvigorated providers become ambassadors for culture change and exemplars for how to conduct bedside rounds in busy clinical settings.

PREPARING A TEAM FOR BEDSIDE ROUNDING

Preparation is essential before teams round at the bedside. The rationale, core principles, evidence base, and necessary skills can be conveyed during orientation sessions. Team leaders benefit from more in-depth seminars where they practice communication skills and try out approaches to teach these skills at the bedside.

Getting buy-in from the rounding team is a critical next step. The following questions prompt teams to explore their concerns and develop a vision for what they hope to accomplish during rounds.

"What Are Your Concerns About Bedside Rounding?"

Getting the team's concerns on the table and listening to them nonjudgmentally builds mutual trust, promotes honesty, and demonstrates respect for diverse opinions.

"What Can Be Learned Best at the Bedside?"

Teams usually list 2 primary educational objectives:

1. Watching senior clinicians demonstrate physical examination maneuvers, and
2. Learning from experienced clinicians about how to approach challenging conversations.[22]

"How Can We Conduct Rounds so That Patients Benefit from the Time We Invest at Their Bedside?"

This question prompts teams to consider how to make rounds that are patient centered as well as patient proximate. This is a good time for the team to discuss relationship-centered communication skills that will elicit what "matters to the patient" in addition to "what's the matter with the patient."[26]

STRATEGIES FOR CONDUCTING BEDSIDE ROUNDS

We approach bedside rounds using the 3-stage process described by Faith Fitzgerald (**Box 1**).[27]

Before the Bedside

In any clinical setting, a key preparatory step is to plan the rounding strategy before embarking. Team leaders assess work volume and decide if the team will see all patients or prioritize those who need urgent attention, new admissions, and potential discharges.

The next step is to set the stage. Patients must be informed ahead of time about what to expect. In a teaching hospital, this is usually done by the learner caring for the patient. On a nonteaching service, the bedside nurse might be the best person to inform the patient.

Specific educational objectives should be reviewed, roles clarified, and expectations established for team function and efficiency. We suggest setting a target of about

---

Box 1
Bedside rounds choreography

Before the Bedside

Prepare the team and get buy-in: What can be learned best at the bedside? How can bedside rounds contribute to patient care?

Set expectations: Positions at the bedside; amount of time for the presentation (5 minutes); total time in the room (15 minutes – can vary based on workflow and objectives); assign who will open the computer and enter orders during rounds; each team member should have a task (eg, critique of the presentation; noticing ICE and PEARLS)

Prepare the patient: Request permission ahead of time; explain the purpose of rounds and what to expect in terms of duration, team size, and teaching; ensure confidentiality.

At the Bedside

Begin well: Introduce the team; have patient introduce visitors; explain purpose; check for patient comfort and minimize distractions; sit if possible; invite patient participation.

Communication pitfalls: Limit medical jargon; use language the patient understands; avoid pejorative labels and practice etiquette; talk with the patient, not just about the patient.

Bedside teaching: Limit the number of teaching points (eg, one each from the history, physical examination, and clinical reasoning); less is usually more; engage all learners; "narrate" the examination while teaching.

PEARLS: Look for opportunities to use at least one of the PEARLS during every patient encounter.

ICE: Inquire about the patient's perspective; also ask, "How has this illness impacted your life?"

Teach Back: Confirm patient understanding: "How will you explain the treatment plan to your family?"

Invite the patient and family to share other concerns, questions, or needs before leaving the room.

After the Bedside:

Check back with the patient: A team member visits the patient later in the day to assess response to rounds and ask about additional concerns or questions.

Debrief and feedback: The team reflects on the interaction, what was learned about the patient, and what skills were demonstrated; patient care tasks are reviewed and assigned.

Abbreviations: ICE, ideas, concerns, expectations; PEARLS, partnership, empathy, apology/appreciation, respect, legitimization, support.
  Adapted from Lichstein PR. Returning to the bedside: notes from a clinical educator. N C Med J 2015;76:174–9; with permission.

---

5 minutes for the bedside patient presentation and a total of about 15 minutes spent at the bedside. Time targets must be flexible depending on workflow demands of the day and service structure. Concise presentations require rehearsal, particularly for medical students who are new to bedside presentations. Decisions about which elements of the history and examination are salient to understanding the patient's clinical presentation and which can be left out are informed by clinical reasoning as well as the time target. Time targets are more easily met as the team gains experience with bedside rounding. It is helpful if the attending physician reviews the chart before bedside rounds so that the encounter is less focused on information transfer and more time is available for patient engagement and teaching.

We suggest that, before entering a patient's room, the team consider the following questions:

- What should we know about this patient before we enter the room?
- Do you have any concerns about presenting at the bedside? Any topics or issues that we should know about before entering?
- What would you like us to focus on during the interaction?
- What elements of the history and/or physical examination would you like us to clarify?
- Do you have any concerns about the patient's or family's response to bedside presentation?

At the Bedside

Bedside choreography

We define "bedside choreography" as a standard rehearsed way in which the team enters the room and convenes around the bedside.[21] The purpose is to set the team up for success in accomplishing its goals in education, patient care, and efficiency. Of course, even the best planned choreography will encounter challenges (eg, the patient is about to leave for a procedure, the intravenous infusion pump is beeping, etc). Flexibility is essential while holding true to patient-centered principles.

Choreography implies that each team member is assigned and knows her or his place at the bedside before the team enters the room. For example, the medical student presenting the case may have an assigned place to the left of the patient with a resident standing next to her. The attending physician may have an assigned place to the right of the patient. Another resident may be in charge of the electronic record and another student may be assigned to critique the presentation at the foot of the bed. The remaining team members may be assigned to observe aspects of the interaction, or demonstrate/practice a physical examination maneuver.

Introductions, etiquette, explanation of purpose, and invitation to participate

First impressions are important.[28,29] Patients and families are particularly attuned to verbal and nonverbal clues when providers enter their room. They can tell within seconds if a provider is in the moment and truly there to care for them. Knock and wait for a response before entering. Warmly greet the patient by name, introduce all members of the team and then ask the patient to introduce all visitors. "Who do you have with you?" and, "Would you like them to stay or would you prefer that they step out until we're done?" Minimize distractions (eg, turn off the TV), attend to patient comfort, and invite the patient to participate. Inform the patient that one clinician will "man the computer" during rounds to access information and enter orders. Whenever possible, sit down. Sitting expands the patient's sense of the duration of the visit. Finding a chair may be challenging in some hospital rooms, but taking a few moments for the presenter and/or attending to sit is worth the effort. Explain the purpose of rounds and what the patient should expect.

Patient presentation and integration of the clinical examination

Presentation at the bedside should follow a standard format with a set time limit. The format will vary based on whether it is a daily update or an initial history and physical. We prefer for presenters to speak directly to their team but also include the patient in the discussion (80% to team; 20% to patient). Some attending physicians prefer to hear a concise 5-minute summary of the patient's entire history and physical examination. Others prefer to pause after presentation of both the history and the physical examination to integrate demonstration of interviewing or physical examination maneuvers before wrapping up with the assessment, plan, and counseling of the patient.

We encourage the presenter to learn something about the patient as a person and begin the bedside presentation by placing the patient in their life context. "Mr Smith is a retired farmer from a small town about 100 miles from here and today he's missing his family and his dogs." A bit of "small talk before big talk" conveys respect and interest in the patient as a person rather than a stranger.

Clinical examination teaching can be integrated into bedside rounding in several ways. Use of strategies such as the Five-Minute Moment from the Stanford Bedside Medicine group can be seamlessly integrated in the context of bedside rounds.[30] In this model, the teaching physician provides historical context on a physical examination maneuver, demonstrates the proper technique and common errors, and discusses the interpretation of the finding. Effective teachers frequently "narrate" the skills they are demonstrating to maintain learner attention and reinforce concepts. The bedside is also an opportunity for direct observation, coaching, and assessment of communication skills and professionalism. The presence of a warm, "covalent bond" between presenter and patient is evidence that attention has been devoted to building a relationship (Jeff Wiese, personal communication, 2017).

Wrapping up the Visit

In keeping with the adage that the first and last 5 minutes of an interaction are best remembered, we suggest investing in the wrap-up before the team exits the room.

- Summarize findings: Statements should be clear, brief, and use language the patient understands. Clarify medical jargon that the patient may not have understood.
- Chunk and check: Information is best delivered and received in manageable "chunks" rather than longer "downloads." Providers should resist the well-intentioned yet ineffective tendency to launch into extensive information "downloads" that patients and families often find overwhelming, especially when cognitive function may be reduced by anxiety, medication, and illness. The key is dialogue rather than monologue. After each chunk of information, check for the patient's understanding, questions, and concerns. Respond to these before proceeding to the next chunk of information. When possible, link information and explanations to the patient's ideas, concerns, and expectations (ie, the "ICE" questions [ideas, concerns, expectations] discussed elsewhere in this article).
- Teach back is an evidence-based approach to assess patient understanding.[31] It asks patients to teach back their understanding of what has been discussed and the plan for the day. Teach back is preferable to reliance on nonverbal clues (head nodding) or answers to questions like, "Do you understand what I've been telling you?" Teach back questions we find helpful are:

"How will you explain things to your family when they call later today?" or, "Doctors aren't always the best at explaining things and it's important that we're on the same page. So, please tell me your understanding of what we've discussed"

- Conclude by asking patient and family, "What other concerns or questions would you like us to address before we leave?" End by expressing partnership, appreciation, and support. Let the patient know which team member will be back to check on them and when.

OTHER PATIENT-CENTERED COMMUNICATION TIPS FOR TEAMS AT THE BEDSIDE

Each encounter provides opportunities to use relationship-centered communication skills to elicit the patient's perspective and respond to her or his emotions. The ICE questions are a good starting point for learning about the patient's perspective (**Box 2**).[32]

Box 2
Patient perspective using ICE questions

Ideas

"Many patients have ideas about the cause of their illness and I'm interested to hear about yours."

"What was your understanding of why your PCP recommended that you be admitted to the hospital?"

Concerns

"What worries you about your illness?"

"What are your concerns (or fears) about being discharged home tomorrow?"

Expectations

"What do you hope we will accomplish during your hospitalization?

Abbreviations: ICE, ideas, concerns, expectations; PCP, primary care provider.

PEARLS: Responding to Patient Emotions

Empathy is conveyed both verbally and nonverbally.[33] PEARLS (partnership, empathy, apology/appreciation, respect, legitimization, support) is a mnemonic for relationship-centered verbal responses developed by the Academy on Communication in Healthcare (**Box 3**).[34] Empathy can be conveyed through a reflective statement followed by a pause allowing time for the patient to respond. Reflections shift the focus of the interview from data gathering to acknowledging emotion. With advanced preparation, providers learn to notice PEARLS opportunities during every bedside visit. Although it is not feasible, or even necessary, to respond to every empathic opportunity, we suggest using at least one of the PEARLS during every bedside encounter. In general, respond to strong patient emotions when they arise. If not, they tend to keep coming up.[35]

After the Bedside

Even 1 or 2 minutes of debriefing after a patient encounter can enhance learning and clarify tasks.[36] Interactions can be debriefed immediately after leaving the patient's room (perhaps in the hallway) or at the end of the day. The following questions help to guide the debrief. Ask team members with observation tasks to give their reports on the interaction. "What PEARLS opportunities did you notice?" "How do you think the patient/family experienced our interaction?" Draw attention to instructive aspects of the interaction by asking, "What did you notice about how I responded when tears welled up in her eyes?" or "How successfully did we address the patient's concerns?" Similar strategies reinforce physical examination skills.

Inquire about any final concerns about the interaction, what was learned, what questions remain, and what issues need to be investigated further. We suggest that one team member returns to the bedside later in the day for a quick assessment of patient and family reactions to bedside rounds.

RETURN TO VIGNETTE 1: THE TEACHING SERVICE

Dr Wells meets with her team on the first day of the rotation to discuss the rationale for bedside rounding and gains buy-in. They discuss the elements of bedside choreography, assign team member roles, and review the presentation format and patient-centered communication tools. After the first few patients, Dr Wells sets her stopwatch

---

Box 3
PEARLS

- Partnership
  "We'll work together on managing your pain."
  "Dr Ellis will be back at 2 PM to talk with you about the results of your MRI."

- Empathy (reflective statement followed by a pause).
  "I can see it's been really difficult not being able to walk for the past several weeks."
  "I can only imagine how complex your life has been."
  "Help me better understand how it's been for you."

- Apology and Appreciation
  "I/we apologize for keeping you waiting. We know you've been anxious to hear the results of your tests."
  "I/we appreciate your patience. Your time is valuable."

- Respect
  "Your thoughts and preferences are important to us."
  "We respect all that you've done to manage these problems on your own."

- Legitimization
  "Many patients get angry when they feel they're not getting answers."
  "Most patients hate being kept NPO."
  "When patients hear different messages from each provider they often wonder if the left hand knows what the right hand is doing."

- Support
  "I will be with you each step of the way."
  "Please let me know what I can do to help you get through this illness."

Abbreviations: NPO, nil per os; PEARLS, partnership, empathy, apology/appreciation, respect, legitimization, support.

---

and finds that the team is able to round on a patient at bedside in 15 minutes, while incorporating focused physical examination teaching. Multiple patients and their family members during the first week of the new process comment on how impressed they are with the work of the teaching team and their appreciation for their time and care at the bedside. Dr Wells and her team approach the leadership of the residency program to discuss implementing bedside rounding as a broader program initiative.

RETURN TO VIGNETTE 2: THE NONTEACHING SERVICE

Dr Johnson approaches the medical and nursing directors of his hospital to discuss the potential benefits of interprofessional bedside rounding.[37] They decide to pilot joint physician and nursing rounds on his primary hospital unit. Within the first week, the nursing staff note that efficiency is improved, important and clinically relevant findings are discussed between Dr Johnson and nurses daily, and patients report that they feel that "everyone is on the same page." After 3 months, patient satisfaction scores increase and hospital leaders are pleased. Dr Johnson is asked by hospital leadership to lead a task force to make joint physician and nursing rounds standard throughout the hospital.

REFERENCES

1. LaCombe MA. On bedside teaching. Ann Intern Med 1997;126(3):217–20.
2. Stickrath D, Noble M, Prochazka A, et al. Attending rounds in the current era: what is and is not happening. JAMA Intern Med 2013;173(12):1084–9. Available at: www.JAMAINTERNALMED.COM.

3. Thayer W. Osler the teacher. Bull Johns Hopkins Hosp 1919;303(30):198–200.

4. William KN, Ramani S, Fraser B, et al. Improving bedside teaching: findings from a focus group study of learners. Acad Med 2008;83(3):257–64.

5. Crumlish CM, Yialamas MA, McMahon GT. Quantification of bedside teaching by an academic hospitalist group. J Hosp Med 2009;4:304–7.

6. Verghese A. Culture shock: patient as icon, icon as patient. N Engl J Med 2008; 359(26):2748–51.

7. Linfors EW, Neelon FA. Sounding boards. The case of bedside rounds. N Engl J Med 1980;303(21):1230–3.

8. Blythe WB. The numbers racket. N C Med J 1988;49:26–7.

9. Gonzalo JD, Kuperman E, Lahman E, et al. Bedside interprofessional rounds: perceptions of benefits and barriers by internal medicine nursing staff, attending physicians and housestaff physicians. J Hosp Med 2014;9:646–51.

10. Block L, Habicht R, Wu AW, et al. In the wake of the 2003 and 2011 duty hours regulations, how do internal medicine interns spend their time? J Gen Intern Med 2013;28(8):1042–7.

11. Thibault GE. Bedside rounds revisited. N Engl J Med 1997;336(16):1174–5.

12. Wang-Chang RM, Barnas GP, Sigmann P, et al. Bedside case presentations: why patients like them but learners don't. J Gen Intern Med 1989;4:284–7.

13. Wachter RM, Verghese A. The attending physician on the wards: finding a new homeostasis. JAMA 2012;308(10):977–8.

14. Lehman LS, Brancati FL, Chen MC, et al. The effect of bedside case presentations on patient's perception of the medical care. N Engl J Med 1997;336:1150–5.

15. Levinson W, Lesser CS, Epstein RM. Developing physician communication skills for patient-centered care. Health Aff 2010;29(7):1310–8.

16. Huang KTL, Minahan J, Brita-Rossi P, et al. All together now: impact of a regionalization and bedside rounding initiative on the efficiency and inclusiveness of clinical rounds. J Hosp Med 2017;12:150–6.

17. Gonzalo JD, Chuang CH, Huang G, et al. The return of bedside rounds: an educational intervention. J Gen Intern Med 2010;25(8):792–8.

18. Levinson W, Gorawara-Bhat R, Lamb J. A study of patient cues and physician responses in primary care and surgical settings. JAMA 2000;284:1021–7.

19. Hojat M, Louis DZ, Markham FW, et al. Physicians' empathy and clinical outcomes for diabetic patients. Acad Med 2011;86:359–64.

20. Gonzalo JD, Heist BS, Duffy BL, et al. The art of bedside rounds: a multi-center qualitative study of strategies used by experienced bedside teachers. J Gen Intern Med 2012;28(3):412–20.

21. Lichstein PR. Returning to the bedside: notes from a clinical educator. N C Med J 2015;76:174–9.

22. Mattern WD, Weinholtz D, Friedman CP. The attending physician as teacher. N Engl J Med 1983;308(19):1129–32.

23. Lesser CS, Lucey CR, Egener B, et al. A behavioral and systems view of professionalism. JAMA 2010;304(24):2732–7.

24. Elder A, Chi J, Ozdalga E, et al. A piece of my mind. The road back to the bedside. JAMA 2013;310(8):799–800.

25. Boissy A, Windover AK, Bokar D, et al. Communication skills training for physicians improves patient satisfaction. J Gen Intern Med 2016;31(7):755–61.

26. Barry MJ, Edgman-Levitan S. Shared decision making — the pinnacle of patient-centered care. N Engl J Med 2012;366:780–1.

27. Fitzgerald FT. Bedside teaching. West J Med 1993;158:418–20.

28. Kahn MW. Etiquette-based medicine. N Engl J Med 2008;358(19):1988–9.

29. Tackett S, Tad-y D, Rios R, et al. Appraising the practice of etiquette-based medicine in the inpatient setting. J Gen Intern Med 2013;28(7):908–13.
30. Chi J, Artandi M, Kugle J, et al. The five-minute moment. Am J Med 2016;129(8): 792–5.
31. Schillinger D, Piette J, Grumbach K, et al. Closing the loop: physician communication with diabetic patients who have low health literacy. Arch Intern Med 2003; 163:83–90.
32. Tate P. Ideas, concerns and expectations. Medicine 2005;33(2):26–7.
33. Riess H, Kraft-Todd G. EMPATHY: a tool to enhance nonverbal communication between clinicians and their patient. Acad Med 2014;89(8):1108–12.
34. Clark W, Hewson M, Fry M, et al. Communication skills reference card. St Louis (MO): American Academy on Communication in Healthcare; 2014.
35. Cole SA, Bird J, Weiner JS. Function one: build the relationship. In: Cole SA, Bird J, editors. The medical interview: the three function approach. 3rd edition. Philadelphia: Saunders; 2014. p. 16–7.
36. Wear D, Zarconi J, Kumagai A, et al. Slow medical education. Acad Med 2015; 90:289–93.
37. Stein J, Murphy DH, Payne C, et al. A remedy for fragmented hospital care. Harvard Business Review 2013.

The Clinical Examination and Socially At-Risk Populations

The Examination Matters for Health Disparities

Karly A. Murphy, MD[a],*, Alejandra Ellison-Barnes, MD[b],
Erica N. Johnson, MD[c], Lisa A. Cooper, MD, MPH[d,e]

KEYWORDS

- Social determinants of health • Health care disparities • Patient-centered care
- Shared decision making • Cultural competency

KEY POINTS

- Disparities exist in health status, health outcomes, and health care delivery.
- The medical interview provides an opportunity for eliciting and addressing the social determinants of health.
- To build a relationship, clinicians should strive to individualize the patient, respond to emotion, and be aware of personal bias/values.
- In gathering data, clinicians may seek information about domains for social risk, and screening tools exist to facilitate this.
- Education, counseling, and decision making should take into account the individual patient's context, health literacy, and degree of activation.

Disclosure Statement: None.
[a] Department of Medicine, Johns Hopkins Hospital, 2024 East Monument Street, Suite 2-500, Baltimore, MD 21287, USA; [b] Osler Medical Residency Training Program, Department of Medicine, Johns Hopkins Hospital, 1800 Orleans Street, Baltimore, MD 21287, USA; [c] Johns Hopkins Bayview Internal Medicine Residency, Department of Medicine, Division of Infectious Diseases, Johns Hopkins University School of Medicine, Johns Hopkins Bayview Medical Center, Mason F. Lord Building, Center Tower Suite 381, 5200 Eastern Avenue, Baltimore, MD 21224, USA; [d] Department of Medicine, Johns Hopkins Center for Health Equity, Johns Hopkins University School, 2024 East Monument Street, Suite 2-500, Baltimore, MD 21287, USA; [e] Department of Health, Behavior and Society, Johns Hopkins Bloomberg School of Public Health, Center for Health Equity, Johns Hopkins University, 2024 East Monument Street, Suite 2-500, Baltimore, MD 21287, USA
* Corresponding author.
E-mail address: kburke34@jhmi.edu

INTRODUCTION

The population of the United States is increasingly diverse. Recent estimates show the US population is 26.4% nonwhite, 13.2% foreign-born, and 3.4% lesbian, gay, bisexual, transgender (LGBT).[1] Economic inequality is also increasing, with the top 1% of the population holding an estimated 42% of the nation's wealth.[2] Sociocultural differences between patients and clinicians can create communication challenges and increase the potential for disparities.[3–5]

There are disparities in health status and health outcomes for many subpopulations.[6] These differences span individual assessments of health status to maternal mortality to morbidity from a myriad of chronic diseases.[3] Increasingly, it is recognized that disparities are driven not by differences in biology or individual patient characteristics, but rather by social determinants, or the conditions of the environments in which people live, including access to healthy food, education, employment, transportation, and housing options.[3,4]

Just as disparities exist in health, there are also disparities in the care people receive when they interface with the health care system. The National Academy of Medicine's (formerly the Institute of Medicine) landmark report *Unequal Treatment* found that members of racial and ethnic minority groups did not always receive needed services at the same rates as whites, and that disparities existed across a range of diseases and persisted even after accounting for confounders such as insurance status and disease severity.[7] Health disparities are also influenced by the social environment, including the quality of interpersonal care, in health care settings.[7,8]

The health care workforce remains less diverse than the US population as a whole. Only about one-third of all physicians are women, and only 8.9% of physicians identify as black or African American, American Indian or Alaska Native, or Hispanic or Latino.[9] Concordance on various dimensions between patients and clinicians, including both visible demographic characteristics and underlying attitudes and values, positively affects the relationship.[8] Racial concordance between patients and providers has been linked to longer clinic visits, more positive patient affect, and greater ratings of patient satisfaction, adherence, and participatory decision making.[10,11] However, such concordance is not always achievable owing to the systemic disparities in the workforce as well as local factors. Even in the best cases, there is rarely full concordance of all aspects of identity between patient and clinician.

The medical interview serves 4 functions: relationship building, data gathering, patient education and counseling, and facilitation and patient activation.[12] We describe how clinicians can uncover and address the social determinants of health within this conceptual framework during a patient–clinician encounter. It is also important for clinicians to consider their relationships with the broader communities in which they work and their relationships with other clinicians.

RELATIONSHIP BUILDING
Dimensions of Relationship-Centered Care

Many studies have reported reduced levels of trust among racial and ethnic minorities in physicians, researchers, and the health care system.[8,13,14] Relationship-centered care considers the experiences, values, and perspectives of the patient and clinician, and how these intersect in the clinical encounter.[7,15] To build a successful patient–clinician relationship, mutual respect, communication, knowing, affiliation/liking, trust, and partnership building must all be present.[8] Respect for the individual underlies and enhances each of these dimensions, and communication is the behavioral action through which the other dimensions are observed and measured.[8,16] To know a person is to be familiar with them as an individual; to like a person is to find the person agreeable, whereas affiliation is to feel a shared sense of identity or purpose.[8] As patients and clinicians know each other better, they build greater trust. Patients trust clinicians who demonstrate trustworthiness through their benevolence, integrity, and competence.[17] Clinically strong partnerships reflect the unique background and opinion of each participant, enable shared decision making, and lead to greater patient satisfaction and engagement.[8,14]

Behaviors of Relationship-Centered Care

Relationship building is a deliberate practice of behaviors that demonstrate emotional support, reassurance, and respect.[12,15] Verbal behaviors explicitly invite an exchange of information. Nonverbal behaviors include a physician's friendliness, eye contact, posture, voice cadence and tone, and level of engagement with gestures and use of touch. The provider's affect, tone, degree of verbal dominance, amount of information provided, and time spent influence communication (**Box 1**).[13]

Racial disparities in communication behaviors have been observed.[13,15–17] African American patients experience less affective behavior and tone and higher percentages of physician dominance compared with Caucasian patients.[13,18] Time spent on mental health topics varies by physician race, and physician-demonstrated empathy varies by patient race.[16] Similarly, African American patients experience less rapport building on topics ranging from mental health to chronic disease management to end-of-life care.[13,17,19,20]

Attitudes Within Relationship-Centered Care

Relationship-centered care also recognizes that patients and clinicians enter into this relationship with opinions and attitudes. Attitudes, as an assumed way of thinking, can arise in response to a repeated stimulus, such as an object or situation. Attitudes become biases when the line of thinking becomes prejudiced against a person or a group.[18]

Medical training often emphasizes population risk factors and objectivity.[13,19] However, these processes can reinforce stereotypes and promote bias.[21] Implicit biases

---

Box 1
Strategies to build rapport and trust

- Individualize the patient.
  - "How would you like me to address you—as Mr/Mrs X, by your first name, or something else?"
  - "Who is important to you? What is important to you?"

- Respond to emotion.
  - Use empathic statements.
  - Legitimize and validate the patient's emotions.
  - Allow for periods of silence.
  - Invite questions.

- Self-reflection
  - Learn about your own implicit biases and values.

- Increase your engagement with the community you serve and/or with persons who differ from you with regard to social or cultural background.

are the unconscious thoughts and feelings, stemming from automatic evaluative processes based on memory and experience.[20,22] Medical providers harbor unconscious biases at the same frequency as the general population.[23–26] Implicit bias influences diagnosis, treatment recommendations, questions asked of the patient, and diagnostic tests ordered.[24]

Bias manifests itself in behaviors that impede relationship building. Physicians with higher levels of general race bias on the implicit association test were more likely to talk slowly, have greater verbal dominance, and have less patient-centered dialogue.[19] In addition, African American patients who interacted with a physician with a higher level of bias were more likely to report lower levels of trust, respect, and engagement in clinical decision making.[19] Strategies to reduce implicit bias should focus on acknowledgment of bias and individualizing the patient.[20,21,23,24] When clinicians know a patient as an individual, it brings them away from stereotyping and cognitive shortcuts and toward mutual partnership.[8]

DATA GATHERING

The history of present illness is the focus of the medical interview, an information exchange designed to lead to a diagnosis. Traditionally, physicians ask questions and receive information through a biomedical or disease-focused lens.[25] This knowledge should be expanded to integrate psychosocial domains, including lifestyle, social context, education, and the patient's perspective of their illness.[25] A pure biomedical line of questioning reflects a physician-dominant voice, which can be at the expense of the patient's perspective.[11]

The National Academy of Science, Engineering, and Medicine has identified 5 domains for social risk: low socioeconomic position, disadvantaged neighborhood, social isolation, racial or ethnic minority status, and lesbian, gay, or bisexual orientation or transgender status. Limited health literacy has also been linked to health disparities; however, it is considered to be more modifiable than the 5 domains listed.[3,26]

These social risk domains influence health outcomes on a personal and systemic level.[4,27] Eliciting these social risk factors provides important data to better understand the patient as a person and to assess home environment, risk for nonadherence, and potential barriers to care and disease self-management. In the United States, adults living below the poverty line are 5 times more likely to report being in poor or fair health as compared with adults who claim incomes at least 4 times the federal poverty line.[26,27] Housing instability, food insecurity, and exposure to violence have been shown to increase health care use.[28,29] Low-income neighborhoods are more likely to have a higher density of fast food and convenience markets, increasing the risk of obesity. Residents who do not have easy access to such ready-made or processed food have lower rates of obesity.[27,30] Lower homicide rates have been observed in neighborhoods in which residents self-rank high levels of mutual trust.[31,32] Racism, particularly structural racism, is another driver of disparities.[33,34]

Although the social history has always been included in clinical interviewing courses, many clinicians may not feel competent how to ask patients about social determinants of health or what to do once that information is obtained. Standardized screening tools have been developed by Health Leads, an organization founded to connect patients to community based resources, and the Centers for Medicare and Medicaid Services, but are not yet part of routine clinical assessment.[28,35] Importantly, a positive screen to any of the questions is actionable.[35] Each survey encompasses 5 health-related social need domains: housing instability, food insecurity, transportation needs, utility needs, and interpersonal safety (**Table 1**). Health Leads also includes a

Table 1
Screening for social risk

Social Need Domain	Examples
Housing instability	Safety of housing, homelessness, inability to pay rent
Food insecurity	Access to nutritious food on a reliable basis
Utility needs	Shut off notices, phone use
Transportation	Access to affordable transportation for medical or public transport
Interpersonal safety	Intimate partner violence, elder abuse, child abuse, community
Financial resource strains	Social security or disability benefits, financial literacy/budgeting, stretching medications owing to cost, difficulty accessing benefits

question on financial resource strains.[28,35] Other social need domains include childcare, education, employment, health behaviors (including smoking, alcohol and substance use), social isolation, and behavioral health. In addition to using screening tools, it is important for clinicians to increase their use of open-ended questions, allowing patients to tell their full stories and elaborate on their concerns. Psychiatrist and anthropologist Arthur Kleinman proposed the use of 8 questions to probe the patient's explanatory model of illness (**Box 2**).[36]

PATIENT EDUCATION AND COUNSELING

When data gathering is expanded to include information about the social determinants of health, the scope of patient education and counseling broadens (**Box 3**). In addition to addressing the direct physical manifestation of illness and the immediate contributors, clinicians can address underlying barriers to achieving health. A clinician might recognize that a patient has limited food options or access to spaces to exercise in their neighborhood, or that the patient faces chronic stress from experiencing racism. Clinicians must become familiar with locally available resources and make referrals to community-based organizations that address social needs, ranging from substance abuse and mental health programs to support groups, to food pantries, job training services, and housing, utility, and prescription assistance programs.

Box 2
Eliciting patient's explanatory model

1. What do you think caused your problem?
2. Why do you think it started when it did?
3. What do you think your sickness does to you?
4. How severe is your sickness? Do you think it will last a long time, or will it be better soon in your opinion?
5. What are the chief problems your sickness has caused for you?
6. What do you fear most about your sickness?
7. What kind of treatment do you think you should receive?
8. What are the most important results you hope to get from treatment?

From Kleinman A, Eisenberg L, Good B. Culture, illness, and care: clinical lessons from anthropological and cross-cultural research. Ann Intern Med 1978;88(2):256; with permission.

> **Box 3**
> **Training opportunities and educational resources**
>
> *Patient education*
>
> - Screen for health literacy using single items.
>   - How often do you need to have someone help you when you read instructions, pamphlets, or other written material from your doctor or pharmacy?
>   - How confident are you filling out medical forms by yourself?
> - Tailor education to individual patient goals.
> - Consider language and literacy barriers.
> - Use the teach-back technique.
> - Learn about local resources.
>
> *Patient activation*
>
> - Engage in patient-centered decision making.
>   - Paraphrase and interpret.
>   - Ask the patient for opinions and suggestions.
>   - Engage in brainstorming options.
>   - Engage in negotiation and joint problem solving.
> - Partner with the patient and the multidisciplinary team.

In providing education and counseling, it is important for clinicians to recall that 14% of adults in the United States cannot read above a basic level.[37] A similar percentage of the population has a less than basic health literacy.[37] Low health literacy is associated with poorer health outcomes, including more frequent hospitalizations and higher mortality rates.[32] Health literacy affects health outcomes through effects on access and use of health care, the patient–provider relationship, and self-management.[31] It is essential to assess literacy and health literacy levels to ensure understanding through the use of nonmedical language and illustrations.[38] There are now single-item screeners for health literacy (see **Box 3**).[39,40] Clinicians should provide information in short, clear statements with opportunities for patients to ask questions. The teach-back technique is useful for confirming patient understanding.[38] Ideally, clinicians frame this technique as a check on their own skills ("I want to make sure I have explained things well"), so that if a patient has difficulty, it is understood to be a reflection of the clinician's deficiency and not the patient's.

Twenty-one percent of Americans sometimes or always speak a language other than English at home; many patients may prefer health information in that language.[1] Among a population of Spanish-speaking patients, when clinicians had higher self-rated language ability and cultural competence, patients were more likely to report better interpersonal processes of care.[41] Similarly, when there was language discordance between patients and clinicians, communication was impeded even when the patients had relatively high health literacy and an interpreter was used.[42] Similar techniques to those used for literacy barriers can be applied when there is a language barrier.

FACILITATION AND PATIENT ACTIVATION

To translate patient education and care plan formulation into improved health outcomes, patients should be involved in decision making and activated to manage their health (see **Box 3**). Patient-centered decision making involves adaptation of the best evidence in medicine to the individual patient context.[43] Short-term health-related outcomes improve when patient context is taken into account in treatment planning.[43] Shared or participatory decision making is a model for clinical interactions in which patients more actively collaborate with their clinicians to formulate care plans that are in line with their preferences and values. Interventions to promote shared decision making increase patient satisfaction across all racial and ethnic groups and improve outcomes for at-risk patients.[44,45]

The concepts of patient engagement, empowerment, and activation can be ambiguous and overlapping. *Engagement* typically refers to the acquisition of motivation to be involved in one's own health care and maintenance. *Empowerment* refers to increasing opportunity for involvement in the decision-making process. *Activation* describes gaining increasing knowledge and skills that allow patients to manage their own health and health care.[46,47] Patients with greater activation are more likely to engage in healthy behaviors and obtain preventive care, and also have biometrics like body mass index and blood pressure within the normal range.[46] Chen and colleagues[48] propose a framework for the development of personalized interventions for the promotion of patient activation that are culturally sensitive. Specifically, patients are at the center of the model—with their personalized knowledge, self-determination, and confidence, and the triad of health providers, community, and health care delivery system encouraging them—resulting in improved health outcomes.[48]

Interventions can increase patient activation in hospital and ambulatory care settings, and across chronic disease management, including for diabetes, hypertension, and mental illness.[46,49] Successful interventions include skill development, problem solving, peer support, change of the social environment, and/or tailored coaching to the individual.[46] For example, patients from predominantly ethnic minority and low-income neighborhoods, who were coached to be more active participants in decisions about their care (and whose physicians were trained in patient-centered interviewing) achieved higher levels of participatory decision making and greater reductions in systolic blood pressure over 12 months compared with patients who were not coached and whose physicians did not receive training. Taking into account patient health literacy is important; in some cases, racial disparities in patient activation can be mediated entirely by health literacy.[44,48]

TRAINING THE CLINICIAN

The National Academy of Medicine recommends training for all clinicians to understand and address the social determinants of health.[5,50] This commitment is viewed as a professional responsibility.[51] Training has focused on cultural competency, emphasizing communication, diagnosis, and management after consideration of a patient's background.[52] More recently, there has been a move toward structural competency, which posits that clinicians be trained to understand how health inequalities are driven by forces at the institutional and societal levels, and to take these factors into account in managing patients.[53] The ecological model, an organizing framework for structural competence, reveals the multiple levels of influence on the health of individual patients (**Fig. 1**).[54]

Learning can be accomplished through traditional didactic sessions or community-based activities.[50,51,55] Training curricula educate health professionals on topics such as structural and cultural competency, community engagement principles, health literacy, and limited English proficiency that are relevant to clinicians (**Table 2**).[56–63]

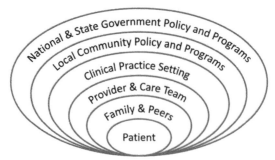

Fig. 1. Ecologic model of multilevel influences on health. (*Adapted from* Mueller M, Purnell TS, Mensah GA, et al. Reducing racial and ethnic disparities in hypertension prevention and control: what will it take to translate research into practice and policy? Am J Hypertens 2015;28(6):700; with permission.)

Community based-teaching can occur through service learning experiences or community-based participatory research.[50] Community-based participatory research is a collaboration between community members, organizations, and researchers with a focus on addressing social, structural, and physical inequity.[64] Guiding principles of community-based participatory research mirror those of relationship-centered care.[8,64]

FUTURE CONSIDERATIONS

Francis Peabody famously wrote, "The secret of the care of the patient is in caring for the patient." In our increasingly diverse and mobile society in which equity is a valued but challenging ideal, clinicians must develop a skillset that allows them to build relationships with patients who might differ from them, deftly gather psychosocial information in the clinical interview, provide relevant education and resources, and facilitate patient activation. In this article, we have introduced concepts and methods relevant to mastering these skills. Beyond the clinical encounter, however, we also encourage physicians to become engaged in efforts to promote equity at the systems level, whether within their institutions, communities, states, or nation, as the social determinants of health exert their influence long before the patient reaches the examination table or hospital bed.

Table 2	
Training opportunities and educational resources	
Meetings and Trainings	Advancing Health Equity in the VA Healthcare system[56]
	Applications of Innovative Methods in Health Equity Research[57]
	Cross Cultural Health Care Program[63]
Curriculum and toolkits	A Train the Trainer Guide: Health Disparities Education[61]
	Caring with Compassion[59]
	Health and Wellbeing for All[60]
	AMA Health Disparities Toolkit[62]
Community-based teaching	Service Learning
	Community-based participatory research
Health outcomes database	County Health Rankings & Roadmaps[55]
Implicit association test	Project Implicit[22]

REFERENCES

1. United States Census Bureau. American FactFinder. Available at: https://factfinder.census.gov/. Accessed August 5, 2017.
2. Saez E, Zucman G. Wealth inequality in the United States since 1913: evidence from capitalized income tax data. Q J Econ 2016;131(2):519–78.
3. Steinwasch DM, Ayanian JZ, Baumgart C, et al. National Academies of Sciences, Engineering, and Medicine, Health and Medicine Division, Board on Health Care Services. Accounting for social risk factors in Medicare payment. Washington, DC: National Academies Press; 2017.
4. Board on Population Health and Public Health Practice Board on Health Care Services, Health and Medicine Division, National Academies of Sciences, Engineering, and Medicine. Systems practices for the care of socially at-risk populations. Washington, DC: National Academies Press; 2016.
5. Lane SD, Delva J, Fisher J, et al. National Academies of Sciences, Engineering, and Medicine. *Accounting for Social Risk Factors in Medicare Payment: Identifying Social Risk Factors*. Washington, DC: The National Academies Press; 2016. Available at: https://doi.org/10.17226/21858.
6. CDC - MMWR - MMWR publications - supplements: past volume. 2013. Available at: https://www.cdc.gov/mmwr/. Accessed August 5, 2017.
7. Smedley BD, Stith AY, Nelson AR, et al. Institute of Medicine. *Unequal Treatment: Confronting Racial and Ethnic Disparities in Health Care*. Washington, DC: The National Academies Press; 2003. Available at: https://doi.org/10.17226/10260.
8. Cooper LA, Beach MC, Johnson RL, et al. Delving below the surface- understanding how race and ethnicity influence relationships in health care. J Gen Intern Med 2006;21(Suppl 1):21.
9. Distribution of physicians by gender. 2017. Available at: http://www.kff.org/other/state-indicator/physicians-by-gender/. Accessed August 5, 2017.
10. Cooper LA, Roter DL, Johnson RL, et al. Patient-centered communication, ratings of care, and concordance of patient and physician race. Ann Intern Med 2003;139(11):907–15.
11. Hall JA, Roter DL, Katz NR. Meta-analysis of correlates of provider behavior in medical encounters. Med Care 1988;26(7):657–75.
12. Roter D. The medical visit context of treatment decision-making and the therapeutic relationship. Health Expect 2000;3(1):17–25.
13. Boulware LE, Cooper LA, Ratner LE, et al. Race and trust in the health care system. Public Health Rep 2003;118(4):358–65.
14. Gordon HS, Street RL Jr, Sharf BF, et al. Racial differences in trust and lung cancer patients' perceptions of physician communication. J Clin Oncol 2006;24(6):904–9.
15. Beach M, Inui T. Relationship-centered care. J Gen Intern Med 2006;21(S1):3–8.
16. Spooner KK, Salemi JL, Salihu HM, et al. Disparities in perceived patient-provider communication quality in the United States: trends and correlates. Patient Educ Couns 2016;99(5):844–54.
17. Schnackenberg AK, Tomlinson EC. Organizational transparency. J Manag 2016;42(7):1784–810.
18. Merriam-Webster. Merriam-Webster web site. 2017. Available at: https://www.merriam-webster.com/. Accessed August 11, 2017.
19. Cooper LA, Roter DL, Carson KA, et al. The associations of clinicians' implicit attitudes about race with medical visit communication and patient ratings of interpersonal care. Am J Public Health 2012;102(5):979–87.

20. Devine PG, Forscher PS, Austin AJ, et al. Long-term reduction in implicit race bias: a prejudice habit-breaking intervention. J Exp Soc Psychol 2012;48(6): 1267–78.

21. Hall WJ, Chapman MV, Lee KM, et al. Implicit racial/ethnic bias among health care professionals and its influence on health care outcomes: a systematic review. Am J Public Health 2015;105(12):60.

22. Education: overview. Project Implicit; 2011. Available at: https://implicit.harvard. edu. Accessed August 9, 2017.

23. Williams DR, Wyatt R. Racial bias in health care and health: challenges and opportunities. JAMA 2015;314(6):555–6.

24. Chapman EN, Kaatz A, Carnes M. Physicians and implicit bias: how doctors may unwittingly perpetuate health care disparities. J Gen Intern Med 2013;28(11): 1504–10.

25. Roter D. The enduring and evolving nature of the patient-physician relationship. Patient Educ Couns 2000;39(1):5–15.

26. Braveman P, Egerter S, Williams DR. The social determinants of health: coming of age. Annu Rev Public Health 2011;32(1):381–98.

27. Woolf SH, Braveman P. Where health disparities begin: the role of social and economic determinants–and why current policies may make matters worse. Health Aff (Millwood) 2011;30(10):1852–9.

28. Billioux A, Verlander K, Anthony S, et al. Standardized screening for health-related social needs in clinical settings. The accountable health communities screening tool. Washington, DC: National Academy of Medicine; 2017.

29. Kushel MB, Vittinghoff E, Haas JS. Factors associated with the health care utilization of homeless persons. JAMA 2001;285(2):200–6.

30. Larson NI, Story MT, Nelson MC. Neighborhood environments: disparities in access to healthy foods in the U.S. Am J Prev Med 2009;36(1):74.

31. Paasche-Orlow MK, Wolf MS. The causal pathways linking health literacy to health outcomes. Am J Health Behav 2007;31(Suppl 1):19.

32. Berkman ND, Sheridan SL, Donahue KE, et al. Low health literacy and health outcomes: an updated systematic review. Ann Intern Med 2011;155(2):97–107.

33. Kozhimannil KB, Medina EM, Hardeman RR. Structural racism and supporting black lives - the role of health professionals. N Engl J Med 2016;375(22):2113.

34. Gee GC, Ford CL. Structural racism and health inequities: old issues, new directions. Du Bois Rev 2011;8(1):115–32.

35. Health leads. Social needs screening toolkit. 2017. Available at: https:// healthleadsusa.org/. Accessed August 3, 2017.

36. Kleinman A, Eisenberg L, Good B. Culture, illness, and care: clinical lessons from anthropologic and cross-cultural research. Ann Intern Med 1978;88(2):251.

37. National assessment of adult literacy (NAAL). Available at: https://nces.ed.gov/. Accessed August 5, 2017.

38. Hersh L, Salzman B, Snyderman D. Health literacy in primary care practice. Am Fam Physician 2015;92(2):118–24. Available at: https://www.aafp.org/afp/2015/ 0715/p118.html. Accessed August 5, 2017.

39. Chew L, Griffin J, Partin M, et al. Validation of screening questions for limited health literacy in a large VA outpatient population. J Gen Intern Med 2008; 23(5):561–6.

40. Morris NS, MacLean CD, Chew LD, et al. The single item literacy screener: evaluation of a brief instrument to identify limited reading ability. BMC Fam Pract 2006;7(1):21.

41. Fernandez A, Schillinger D, Grumbach K, et al. Physician language ability and cultural competence. An exploratory study of communication with Spanish-speaking patients. J Gen Intern Med 2004;19(2):167–74.

42. Sudore RL, Landefeld CS, Pérez-Stable EJ, et al. Unraveling the relationship between literacy, language proficiency, and patient-physician communication. Patient Educ Couns 2009;75(3):398–402.

43. Weiner SJ, Schwartz A, Sharma G, et al. Patient-centered decision making and health care outcomes: an observational study. Ann Intern Med 2013;158(8): 573–9.

44. Cooper L, Roter D, Carson K, et al. A randomized trial to improve patient-centered care and hypertension control in underserved primary care patients. J Gen Intern Med 2011;26(11):1297–304.

45. Durand MA, Carpenter L, Dolan H, et al. Do interventions designed to support shared decision-making reduce health inequalities? A systematic review and meta-analysis. PLoS One 2014;9(4):e94670.

46. Hibbard JH, Greene J. What the evidence shows about patient activation: better health outcomes and care experiences; fewer data on costs. Health Aff (Millwood) 2013;32(2):207–14.

47. Fumagalli LP, Radaelli G, Lettieri E, et al. Patient empowerment and its neighbours: clarifying the boundaries and their mutual relationships. Health Policy 2015;119(3):384–94.

48. Chen J, Mullins CD, Novak P, et al. Personalized strategies to activate and empower patients in health care and reduce health disparities. Health Educ Behav 2016;43(1):25–34.

49. Lubetkin EI, Lu WH, Gold MR. Levels and correlates of patient activation in health center settings: building strategies for improving health outcomes. J Health Care Poor Underserved 2010;21(3):796–808.

50. Cené CW, Peek ME, Jacobs E, et al. Community-based teaching about health disparities: combining education, scholarship, and community service. J Gen Intern Med 2010;25(S2):130–5.

51. Smith WR, Betancourt JR, Wynia MK, et al. Recommendations for teaching about racial and ethnic disparities in health and health care. Ann Intern Med 2007; 147(9):654.

52. Cooper LA, Roter DL. Patient-provider Communication: the effect of race and ethnicity on process and outcomes of health care. In: Smedley BD, Stith AY, Nelson AR, editors. *Unequal Treatment: Confronting Racial and Ethnic Disparities in Health Care*. Institute of Medicine (US) Committee on Understanding and Eliminating Racial and Ethnic Disparities in Health Care. Washington, DC: National Academies Press; 2009. p. 552–93.

53. Wear D, Zarconi J, Aultman JM, et al. Remembering Freddie Gray: medical education for social justice. Acad Med 2017;92(3):312–7.

54. Mueller M, Purnell TS, Mensah GA, et al. Reducing racial and ethnic disparities in hypertension prevention and control: what will it take to translate research into practice and policy? Am J Hypertens 2015;28(6):699–716.

55. Health is where we live. County health rankings & roadmaps web site. 2017. Available at: http://www.countyhealthrankings.org/. Accessed August 11, 2017.

56. Center for Health Equity Research and Promotion. Advancing health equity in the VA healthcare system. Washington, DC: U.S. Department of Veterans Affairs; 2016. Available at: https://www.cherp.research.va.gov/. Accessed August 11, 2017.

57. Johns Hopkins Bloomberg School of Public Health (JHSPH). Applications of innovative methods in health equity research. Johns Hopkins Bloomberg School of Public Health; Available at: https://www.jhsph.edu/courses/. Accessed August 10, 2017.

58. Golden S, Purnell T, Halbert J, et al. A community-engaged cardiovascular health disparities research training curriculum: implementation and preliminary outcomes. Acad Med 2014;89(10):1348–56.

59. Chick DA, Bigelow A, Rye H, et al. Caring with compassion. Ann Arbor (MI): University of Michigan Medical School; 2014. Available at: https://caringwithcompassion.org//. Accessed August 6, 2017.

60. CDC Foundation. Health and well-being for all. Health in a box resources. 2017. Available at: http://www.cdcfoundation.org/. Accessed August 8, 2017.

61. Society of General Internal Medicine. A train the trainer guide: health disparities education. SGIM resource library: education resources. Available at: http://www.sgim.org/. Accessed August 11, 2017.

62. AMA. Reducing disparities in health care. Chicago (IL): American Medical Association; 2017. Available at: www.ama-assn.org/. Accessed August 11, 2017.

63. CCHCP. Equity and inclusion programs. Seattle (WA): The Cross Cultural Health Care Program; 2017. Available at: http://xculture.org/cultural-competency-programs/. Accessed August 11, 2017.

64. Israel BA, Schulz AJ, Parker EA, et al. Review of community-based research: assessing partnership approaches to improve public health. Annu Rev Public Health 1998;19(1):173–202.

Clinical Examination Component of Telemedicine, Telehealth, mHealth, and Connected Health Medical Practices

Ronald S. Weinstein, MD[a],*, Elizabeth A. Krupinski, PhD[b],
Charles R. Doarn, MBA[c]

KEYWORDS

- Telemedicine • Telehealth • mHealth • eHealth • Connected health
- Direct-to-consumer telehealth care

KEY POINTS

- Telemedicine and telehealth involves performing several clinical tests on patients at a distance.
- Video conferencing is often used for telemedicine clinical examinations.
- Many clinical tests are performed at a distance using special medical devices referred to as telemedicine peripherals (eg, electronic stethoscopes, tele-ophthalmoscopes, video-otoscopes, and so forth).
- Telemedicine peripherals can expand and enhance some clinical examinations and, in the future, may even become the standard of care for in-person clinical encounters.
- Some conventional clinical examination tests, such as palpation of the liver, are not currently amenable to telemedicine.

INTRODUCTION

A century ago, the great academic physicians of the day achieved fame based on their remarkable bedside diagnostic skills.[1] These observation-based clinical examination

Disclosure Statement: Dr R.S. Weinstein is on the Advisory Board of GlobalMed. He is not compensated and has no equity interest in GlobalMed. Dr E.A. Krupinski and Mr C.R. Doarn have nothing to disclose.
[a] Arizona Telemedicine Program, University of Arizona College of Medicine, 1501 North Campbell Avenue, Tucson, AZ 85724, USA; [b] Department of Radiology and Imaging Sciences, Emory University, 1364 Clifton Road Northeast D107, Atlanta, GA 30322, USA; [c] Department of Family and Community Medicine, University of Cincinnati, 231 Albert Sabin Way, Cincinnati, OH 45267-0582, USA
* Corresponding author.
E-mail address: rweinstein@telemedicine.arizona.edu

tests (or signs) often bore the names of their creators[2(P650)] and became standard components of in-person clinical examinations. In the twenty-first century, many of these tests can be performed at a distance through telemedicine.[3–7]

Traditional in-person clinical examination tests and their telemedicine counterparts have similar performance characteristics.[3–10] In some clinical settings, the conventional examination's performance might even be improved by integrating a telemedicine peripheral, such as an electronic stethoscope, to aid in data acquisition and interpretation.

Evolution of Telemedicine, Telehealth, eHealth, and Direct-to-Consumer Telehealth Clinical Practices

Teleradiology and tele-psychiatry were among the earliest telemedicine applications. Although the roots of telemedicine date quite far back, the modern era of telemedicine[11] started in 1968, when the Massachusetts General Hospital (MGH) bundled these and other services together into the first hospital-based multispecialty telemedicine practice that offered remote clinical examinations to travelers and airport workers at Logan International Airport. An assortment of ill airline passengers in transit and largely healthy airport workers needing annual physical examinations entered the MGH telemedicine system near gate 23 at the airport. The MGH tele-physicians were stationed 2.7 miles away near the MGH side of the Callahan Tunnel that linked the airport to downtown Boston.[12] Over the next decade, more than 1000 patients received telemedicine clinical examinations through the MGH service. This effort was a high-profile endeavor that had visibility in popular US magazines (**Fig. 1**) and inspired dozens of telemedicine programs around the world.[12]

For unclear reasons, most of these programs disappeared by 1980, leading to a decade hiatus in telemedicine activities. The telemedicine industry was jump-started again in the early 1990s and has undergone continuous growth and refinement in terms of implementation and practice as well as development of a taxonomy framework for research.[12,13] The reasons for this rebound are multidimensional; but some of the key factors include the development and rapid expansion of the Internet, increase in digital communication technologies (especially the smartphone), and, more recently, the reduction in the cost of technologies that drive telemedicine innovations.

Millions of patients around the world have received telemedicine and telehealth services from thousands of providers. In recent years, investments in start-up telemedicine service companies have skyrocketed. Thousands of hospitals are outsourcing selected gap services (eg, nighttime and weekend coverage by teleradiology) and urgent services (eg, tele-stroke services).[4] Direct-to-consumer telemedicine and telehealth services are a more recent entrant into the marketplace. The direct-to-consumer market includes in-store telehealth-enabled primary care services, typically delivered at pharmacies or big box stores; walk-in clinics; as well as services delivered directly to patients through the Internet or mobile devices. Typically, these patient-targeted services deliver a defined set of primary care services directly to patients, at the venue of their choice, and at low, fixed prices. Some evidence suggests that direct-to-consumer telehealth may increase utilization and health care spending by increasing access and convenience. A recent review[14] analyzed commercial claims data from more than 300,000 patients over a 3-year period on direct-to-consumer utilization and spending for acute respiratory illnesses. Ironically, the actual per-episode cost of a telehealth visit was lower than a comparable in-person visit; but the overall convenience resulted in greater use of care, thus, overall making telemedicine potentially more costly. It is important to note that this study did not examine the long-term impact of telemedicine, which might, for example, reduce more expensive health care

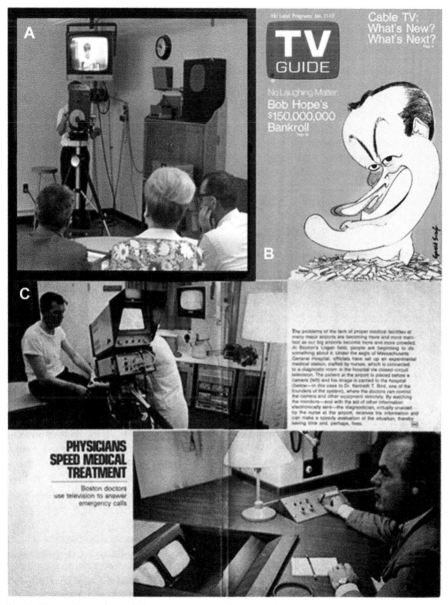

Fig. 1. Pioneering telemedicine programs in the United States. First telemedicine application, a tele-psychiatry service, was established in 1959 by Cecil L. Wittson, MD, the future Dean of the University of Nebraska College of Medicine, in Omaha, Nebraska. (*A*) It linked the Norfolk State Hospital (*television monitor*) to the Nebraska Psychiatric Institute (*foreground*) in Omaha, 112 miles away. The program was in operation for a decade when federal funding ended. Telemedicine was also used to facilitate the transfer of mentally challenged patients. The first complete prototype telemedicine system became operational between the MGH and Logan International Airport in Boston in 1968. (*B*) Historical telemedicine magazine article. Cover of the January 11, 1969 *TV Guide*, "Bob Hope's 65th Birthday" issue: *TV Guide* telemedicine article. (*C*) 2-page spread in 1969 TV Guide. Dr. Kenneth Bird, at the MGH (*lower right*) is remotely controlling, with his right hand, the large movable and

utilization, such as emergency department visits and hospitalizations, because of earlier recognition and treatment of disease.

Telehealth Facilities

In the more recent decades of the modern telemedicine era (1995–2015), many telemedicine clinical encounters originated in dual-purpose outpatient telemedicine clinics operated within rural hospitals, community health centers, or correctional facilities. In order to create these telemedicine clinics, a standard outpatient clinic was often retrofitted into a hybrid standard clinic/telemedicine clinic by outfitting the clinic with a standard videoconferencing setup and adding a mobile telemedicine cart designed to help manage an array of telemedicine peripherals that are plugged into the cart (**Fig. 2**). These mobile carts support 1 or 2 adjustable eye-level video monitors attached to a vertical support post. The carts are ergonomically designed for comfortable face-to-face videoconferencing between the tele-consultant, the patients, and their local case presenter. In addition, there are plug-in ports and lockable storage compartments for telemedicine peripherals.[15]

Telehealth and the Personal Health Care Space

The telemedicine landscape may be shifting away from dedicated telemedicine clinics to individual patient's mobile health and personal health care space at work or at home. The widespread availability of the Internet, ready access to Internet-enabled computing devices, and evolving computer literacy in the general population have facilitated the transition to Web 2.0 technologies.

Smartphones are becoming the next-generation telehealth workstations.[16] Several medical and laboratory services use smartphones attached to relatively inexpensive telehealth accessories, such as blood glucose monitors and electrocardiogram devices.[16] Uses of these technologies are accompanied by an increase in patients' self-performed clinical examinations. Such clinical examinations may be carried out synchronously, under the direct supervision of a distant physician or nurse practitioner, or asynchronously, with the test results reviewed offline at a later time. Often, call support centers are staffed with advanced practice nurses, under the supervision of a physician. In addition to remote health consultations, many health systems post medical results on personalized Web-based portals, which may include some dashboard metrics and analytics to help patients understand their health challenges and potential solutions and to visualize trends in their health status.

Telemedicine Examination Medical Devices (Peripherals)

The special medical examination tools used to conduct a clinical examination at a distance were traditionally called *telemedicine peripherals* (**Fig. 3**A and 3C). This term is a carryover from earlier times when the data streams from telemedicine peripherals were outside the main stream of telecommunications data generated during ordinary videoconferencing. Each of these medical devices now pushes a data stream through a shared digital interface for review by the distant provider.

---

adjustable television camera (*upper left photo*) in the Logan Airport telemedicine clinic, 2.7 miles away. Dr. Bird is focusing the TV camera on the remote patient's left foot's hemorrhagic lesions. The patient's left leg was edited out by the magazine. (*Courtesy of [A]* the McGovern Historical Center, Texas Medical Center Library, IC077 Medical World News Photograph Collection; and *[B, C]* Sai Saha, *TV Guide* magazine.)

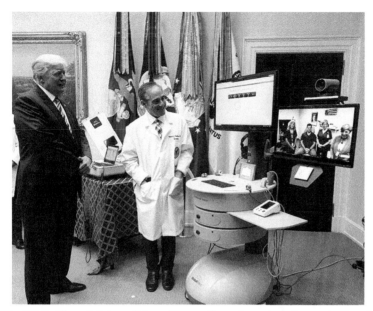

Fig. 2. The White House's telemedicine videoconferencing setup demonstration for President Donald J. Trump by the Secretary of Veterans Affairs (VA), David J. Shulkin, MD (*center*), on August 3, 2017. The light gray mobile telemedicine cart (equipped with 2 video monitors) is designed to help manage an array of telemedicine peripherals (eg, telemedicine clinical examination devices) that are plugged into, and tethered by, the cart. This same model of telemedicine cart is being deployed at VA hospitals and many VA clinics throughout the United States. The president is conversing with a tele-dermatology patient (*video screen, seated*) at a VA clinic in Grants Pass, Oregon. The White House, Air Force One, and Camp David are all equipped for telemedicine. A briefcase-sized miniaturized telemedicine workstation, the type of portable telemedicine workstation carried on both the President's Air Force One and Marine One aircrafts, is visible on the table behind the President and the Secretary of Veterans Affairs. (*Photo courtesy of* GlobalMed and the White House.)

Telemedicine peripherals are evaluated as medical devices and classified as such by the US Food and Drug Administration (FDA), following rigorous evaluation. Generally, the methodological quality of studies of diagnostic tests lags behind the quality of studies of therapeutic interventions.[17,18] This circumstance is due, in part, to the rapid development of technologies and perpetual software upgrades.

The following sections briefly summarize the telemedicine and telehealth patient examination tools most frequently used for telemedicine clinical examinations today.

Videoconference system-based patient clinical examinations
Many telemedicine cases can be handled by standard secure videoconferencing, without using any telemedicine peripherals (**Fig. 3**B).[19,20] In fact, one of the most common telemedicine applications, tele-psychiatry, is typically done by videoconferencing alone.

At the other end of the spectrum, there are clinical settings in which telemedicine workups are technically more complex and require a coordinated team effort at both ends of the encounter in order to be successful. For example, patients with Parkinson disease are ordinarily assessed using a set of neurologic tests that are performed by an experienced provider at the bedside.[21,22] The Unified Parkinson's Disease Rating Scale (UPDRS) was created specifically for telemedicine.[22] The

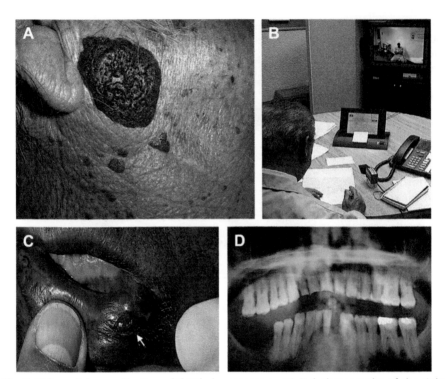

Fig. 3. Telemedicine applications. (*A*) Teledermatoscopy. Digital photography of the right side of a patient's face, with multiple pigmented seborrheic keratosis lesions. (*B*) Corrections telemedicine. A deidentified patient (*on screen*) is shown on the video monitor. The tele-physician is in the foreground noting the patient's history in his medical chart. (*C*) Example of an image captured with a handheld patient examination camera. There is a small nodular lesion of the buccal mucosa (*white arrow*) and adjacent hyperemia. (*D*) Oral teleradiology. Tele-dentistry has been successfully used in Arizona corrections facilities.

UPDRS is a rating tool that follows the longitudinal course of Parkinson disease. It is based on visual impressions only and has been shown to be reliable and valid. This approach to protocol development may be applicable to other disease assessments, but such applications will require validation on a disease-by-disease basis.

General patient examination camera

The telemedicine general patient examination camera is a handheld digital camera plugged into the telemedicine cart. It is equipped with special features designed to augment patient examinations. The general patient examination camera includes specialized lenses, selectable light sources, distance gauges, and built-in digital image capture and video signal outputs. General examination cameras can be used in combination with either asynchronous or synchronous videoconferencing. These general examination cameras provide distant clinicians with optimally illuminated, high-resolution views of selected fields of interest of patients' bodies (**Fig. 3**C). High-end models of these digital cameras can function as an otoscope, nasopharyngoscope, ophthalmoscope, dermatoscope, and a video camera.

Electronic stethoscope

Electronic stethoscopes have several innovative features previously unavailable on conventional acoustic stethoscopes. These features include electronic sound amplification, recording, playback, and even graphic visualization of auscultated sounds. Digitized auscultation data can be transmitted to specialists for interpretation. Live and recorded auscultations can also be streamed simultaneously across multiple wireless stethoscopes for group clinical decision-making and didactics.[23,24] An additional benefit is the high-quality amplification of faint or difficult-to-interpret sounds, which is an especially valuable feature for hearing-impaired physicians.

Tele-ophthalmoscope

Tele-ophthalmoscopes offer features beyond those of traditional ophthalmoscopes. The optics make it easier for the examiner to view intraocular structures at higher magnifications and through an undilated pupil. The integrated digital camera captures high-resolution images at 30 frames per second for real-time imaging. Digital images can be used for immediate diagnosis or stored for asynchronous diagnosis and digital analysis. The wider field of view allows the examiner to more easily explore and document intraocular conditions, including papilledema, diabetic retinopathy, and hypertension.[25–27]

A second category of the ophthalmoscope is the freestanding retinal digital imaging device. These devices are most frequently used for screening of patients for diabetic retinopathy.

Video-otoscope

A standard otoscope provides clinicians with an illuminated and magnified view of the ear canal. A video-otoscope reproduces the otoscope visual field with enhanced viewing capabilities for the nonexpert and at high resolution for the expert. The video-otoscope's visual fields are seen on a local video display as well as at the distant telemedicine consultant's site. Today, some video-otoscopes include built-in digital image capture as well as video recording and playback capabilities.[28,29]

Electronic dermatoscope

Tele-dermatoscopes have integral light sources and magnification lenses to aid visual examination of patients' skin lesions (see **Fig. 3**A). Relatively inexpensive, single-purpose dermatoscopes, not adaptable to other functions, are also available.[30–32] Dermatoscope applications (apps) also exist to support patients and clinicians. The absence of a palpation feature (ie, the ability to assess the firmness or depth of a lesion) is a limitation in some cases.

Digital-endoscope

A digital endoscope is a capsule-size video camera that patients swallow. It images the interior of the bowel as it moves through the gastrointestinal track. The on-board digital camera wirelessly transmits a stream of images to a server for gastroenterologist interpretation.[33]

Electronic scale

A simple, high-yield, telemedicine encounter involves patients with congestive heart failure (CHF) at home, equipped with an electronic scale that transmits daily body weights to a call center. Typically, patients with CHF step on a wireless electronic scale, which measures and transmits their body weight to a nurse's dashboard at a telehealth center. An increase in body weight exceeding a predetermined critical value triggers an instruction to increase the dosage of a diuretic in a predetermined amount. Electronically tracking CHF patient's electronic body weights has reduced hospital readmissions for many patients, saving millions of dollars in health care expenses.[23,34]

Smartphone

The smartphone is playing an increasing role in telemedicine and telehealth. The FDA is fast-tracking approval of both medical apps and mobile medical devices. Today, test-specific medical device-equipped smartphones can be used to perform and analyze an electrocardiogram, conduct an ultrasound scan on patients' hearts, perform clinical ophthalmic examinations, and even measure blood oxygen levels. With other relatively inexpensive accessories, smartphones can be used to evaluate pulmonary function, make breathalyzer measurements, and perform scans of the aorta. In the neurology arena, apps are being developed that may revolutionize migraine headache diagnostics and patient performances with Alzheimer disease or other dementias. The use of smartphones for diagnosing ischemic and hemorrhagic strokes has been validated.[35–39]

Wearables

Wearable devices are widely used to monitor various body functions and activities.[23,34,40(P8)] It is important to note that many consumer-grade wearables may not yield data of clinical diagnostic value as compared with physician-prescribed medical-grade wearables.

Telemedicine Presenter/Site Coordinator

The case coordinator and case presenter are critical members of the telemedicine team at rural sites and in community health centers. The same person may fill both professional roles. The case coordinator aggregates patient information, including the electronic health record, and submits it to the physician or nurse at the distant site. The case presenter serves as the distant clinician's proxy for hands-on examinations and could be a primary care physician, advanced practice nurse, physician assistant, or a nurse.

Limitations of Telemedicine

There are several limitations of telemedicine, some of which are amenable to workarounds. As mentioned earlier, certain clinical applications, such as performing a remote neurology examination, require the teaming of the health worker at the spoke site with the diagnosing physician or advanced nurse practitioner at the telemedicine diagnostic hub.

The telemedicine clinical examination is somewhat limited by the inability of the remote physician to palpate patients. Although imaging can substitute for palpation in certain instances, there are some parts of the physical examination that require direct touch. Technologies are being developed to allow the remote provider to sense palpation in a virtual-reality setting. Ultrasound is an alternative means to obtain the information that palpation provides.[41] Other types of remote palpation systems are being developed, such as wearable haptic systems for the hand and fingertips.[42,43] Tele-robotic surgery, although technically possible, is encumbered with ethical, communications, reliability, and delay issues.

Outcomes and Evidence

There is a large literature on telemedicine published in a select set of dedicated telemedicine journals. Publication of clinical telemedicine articles in leading journals, such as the New England Journal of Medicine and the Journal of the American Medical Association, is relatively uncommon but increasing each year. It should be noted that several trials are reported in the literature that incorporate new telemedicine technologies but do not directly refer to them as telemedicine or telehealth. Nevertheless, there is a general perception in the health care industry that telemedicine is only beginning to enter the mainstream.

Published standards and guidelines represent expert consensus on the current state of medical diagnostic tests, procedures, and even therapies delivered via telemedicine techniques and technologies. The American Telemedicine Association posts authoritative clinical standards and guidelines that are valuable guides to some of the most important service areas in the telemedicine and telehealth industries.[44]

FUTURE CONSIDERATIONS AND SUMMARY

Important factors driving the telemedicine sector forward at an accelerating rate are patient needs for access to care and cost savings at both the patient and health care system levels. There have been numerous studies on the issue of cost in telemedicine, with conflicting results. It is important when reviewing these studies to assess exactly what type of cost analysis was conducted (eg, cost-utility, cost-benefit, cost-effectiveness), what patient population was used, and what costs were included.[45]

Increasingly, hospitals are using commercial clinical service providers that handle a suite of telemedicine services. For example, a teleradiology service company can interpret plain film bone and chest radiographic images, ultrasound, mammography, computerized tomography, and MRI and provide video consultation. Telecardiology services include interpretation of cardiac rhythms and other studies, such as echocardiography, vascular, and nuclear medicine. They also include video consults. Many hospitals are also using tele–intensive-care-unit services that monitor patients 24 hours per day and alert on-site health care providers about emerging problems. These telemedicine services allow hospitals in rural areas to keep patients on-site and with their families, which can also reduce the overall cost.

Today, many private practices and health care systems are becoming hybrid health care providers, presenting their patients with the option to see their medical provider either by telemedicine or in person and scheduling their appointments on-line at the patients' convenience. These private practices will soon be competing with many commercial telehealth service providers that effectively and efficiently manage and transfer patients between physicians and advanced practice nurses and other contract providers who are housed in virtual call centers. Often, these companies have thousands of telehealth workers on-call who hold multiple state licenses and practice in multiple time zones every day.

In addition to legal, regulatory, and reimbursement issues, other significant issues include concerns over the increasing fragmentation of health care services, the slow (but increasing) rate of acceptance of telemedicine by physicians and other key decision makers, and the need for champions of telemedicine to drive acceptance forward. Several systematic reviews of the literature support the effectiveness of telemedicine in numerous clinical specialties.[3–7,46–50]

REFERENCES

1. Sood S, Jugoo S, Dooky R, et al. What is telemedicine?: 104 peer-reviewed perspectives and theoretical underpinnings. Telemed J E Health 2007;13(5):573–90.
2. Jarvis C. Physical examination & health assessment. 7th edition. Elsevier; 2016.
3. Wootton R. Twenty years of telemedicine in chronic disease management-an evidence synthesis. J Telemed Telecare 2012;18:211–20.
4. Weinstein RS, Lopez AM, Joseph BA, et al. Telemedicine, telehealth, and mobile health applications that work: opportunities and barriers. Am J Med 2014;127(3): 183–7.

5. Bashshur RL, Shannon G, Krupinski EA, et al. Sustaining and realizing the promise of telemedicine. Telemed J E Health 2013;19(5):339–45.

6. Bashshur RL, Howell JD, Krupinski EA, et al. The empirical foundations of telemedicine intervention in primary care. Telemed J E Health 2016;22(5):342–75.

7. Bashshur RL, Shannon GW, Smith BR, et al. The empirical foundations of telemedicine interventions for chronic disease management. Telemed J E Health 2014;20(9):769–800.

8. Quinn GE, Ying GS, Daniel E, et al. Validity of a telemedicine system for the evaluation of acute-phase retinopathy of prematurity. JAMA Ophthalmol 2014; 132(10):1178–84.

9. Yager PH, Clark ME, Dapul HR, et al. Reliability of circulatory and neurologic examination by telemedicine in a pediatric intensive care unit. J Pediatr 2014; 165(5):962–6.

10. Siew L, Hsiao A, McCarthy P, et al. Reliability of telemedicine in the assessment of seriously ill children. Pediatrics 2016;137:e20150712.

11. Mermelstein H, Guzman E, Rabinowitz T, et al. The application of technology to health: the evolution of telephone to telemedicine and telepsychiatry: a historical review and look at human factors. J Technol Behav Sci 2017. https://doi.org/10.1007/s41347-017-0010-x.

12. Bashshur RL, Shannon GW. History of telemedicine. New York: Mary Ann Liebert Inc; 2009.

13. Bashshur R, Shannon GW, Krupinski E, et al. The taxonomy of telemedicine. Telemed J E Health 2011;17(6):484–94.

14. Ashwood JS, Mehrotra A, Cowling D, et al. Direct-to-consumer telehealth may increase access to care but does not decrease spending. Health Aff 2017;36(3): 485–91.

15. Powell RE, Henstenburg JM, Cooper G, et al. Patient perceptions of telehealth primary care video visits. Ann Fam Med 2017;15(3):225–9.

16. Dorsey ER, Topol EJ. State of telehealth. N Engl J Med 2016;375(2):154–61.

17. Tatsioni A, Zarin DA, Aronson N, et al. Challenges in systematic reviews of diagnostic technologies. Ann Intern Med 2005;142(12 Pt2):1048–55.

18. Deeks JJ, Bossuyt PM, Gatsonis C. Cochrane handbook for systematic reviews of diagnostic test accuracy, version 0.9 [on-line]. The Cochrane Collaboration; 2016.

19. LeRouge C, Garfield MJ, Hevner AR. Quality attributes in telemedicine video conferencing. In Proceedings of the Annual Hawaii International Conference on System Sciences. IEEE Computer Society 2002;2050–9.

20. Daniel H, Snyder Sulmasy L. Policy recommendations to guide the use of telemedicine in primary cares: an American College of Physicians position paper. Ann Intern Med 2015;163(10):787–9.

21. Durner G, Durner J, Dunsche H, et al. 24/7 Live stream telemedicine home treatment service for Parkinson's disease patients. Mov Disord Clin Pract 2017;4(3): 368–73.

22. Abdolahi A, Scoglio N, Killoran A, et al. Potential reliability and validity of a modified version of the Unified Parkinson's Disease Rating Scale that could be administered remotely. Parkinsonism Relat Disord 2013;19:218–21.

23. Bashi N, Karunanithi M, Fatehi F, et al. Remote monitoring of patients with heart failure: an overview of systematic reviews. J Med Internet Res 2017;19(1):e18.

24. Satou GM, Rheunan H, Alverson D, et al. Telemedicine in pediatric cardiology: a scientific statement from the American Heart Association. Circulation 2017; 135(11):e648–78.

25. Fierson WM, Capone A Jr. Telemedicine for evaluation of retinopathy of prematurity. Pediatrics 2015;135(1):e238–54.
26. Ryan MC, Ostmo S, Jonas K, et al. Development and evaluation of reference standards for image-based telemedicine diagnosis and clinical research studies in ophthalmology. AMIA Annu Symp Proc 2014;2014:1902–10.
27. Rathi S, Tsui E, Mehta N, et al. The current state of teleophthalmology in the United States. Ophthalmology 2017;124(12):1729–34.
28. Biagio L, Swanepoel DW, Adeyemo A, et al. Asynchronous video-otoscopy with a telehealth facilitator. Telemed J E Health 2013;19(4):252–8.
29. Lundberg T, de Jager LB, Laurent C. Diagnostic accuracy of a general practitioner with video-otoscopy collected by a health care facilitator compared to traditional otoscopy. Int J Pediatr Otorhinolaryngol 2017;99:49–53.
30. Krupinski E, Burdick A, Pak H, et al. American Telemedicine Association's practice guidelines for teledermatology. Telemed J E Health 2008;14(3):289–302.
31. Wolf JA, Moreau JF, Akilov O, et al. Diagnostic inaccuracy of smartphone applications for melanoma detection. JAMA Dermatol 2013;149(4):422–6.
32. Ferrandiz L, Ojeda-Vila T, Corrales A, et al. Internet-based skin cancer screening using clinical images alone or in conjunction with dermoscopic images: a randomized teledermoscopy trial. J Am Acad Dermatol 2017;76(4):676–82.
33. Ohta H, Kawashima M. Technical feasibility of patient-friendly screening and treatment of digestive disease by remote control robotic capsule endoscopes via the Internet. Conf Proc IEEE Eng Med Biol Soc 2014;2014:7001–4.
34. Vegesna A, Tran M, Angelaccio M, et al. Remote patient monitoring via non-invasive digital technologies: a systematic review. Telemed J E Health 2017; 23(1):3–17.
35. FDA issues final guidance on mobile medical apps. Available at: http://www.fda.gov/NewsEvents/Newsroom/PressAnnouncements/ucm369431.htm. Accessed September 23, 2013.
36. McCormack M. Medical apps: to regulate, or not to regulate? Available at: http://profitable-practice.softwareadvice.com/medical-apps-to-regulate-or-not-to-regulate-0713/. Accessed September 5, 2013.
37. Bedinger M. Patients lead the way as medicine grapples with apps. Available at: http://www.kaiserhealthnews.org/Stories/2013/June/18/doctors-patients-smartphone-apps.aspx. Accessed August 17, 2017.
38. Versel N. Eric Topol on NBC's rock center. Available at: http://www.youtube.com/watch?v=0B-jUOOrtks. Accessed August 17, 2017.
39. Zangbar B, Pandit V, Rhee P, et al. Smartphone surgery: how technology can transform practice. Telemed J E Health 2014;20(6):590–2.
40. Moore Q, Johnson A. US Health Care Technologies, Center for HEALTH + BIO-SCIENCES. Rice University's Baker Institute for Public Policy; 2015.
41. Young HM, Nesbitt TS. Increasing the capacity of primary care through enabling technology. J Gen Intern Med 2017;32(4):398–403.
42. Campisano F, Ozel S, Ramakrishnan A, et al. Toward a soft robotic skin for autonomous tissue palpation. IIEEE Trans Robot Automation ICRA 2017;6150–5.
43. Pacchierotti C, Sinclair S, Solazzi M, et al. Wearable haptic systems for the fingertip and the hand: taxonomy, review, and perspectives. IEEE Trans Haptics 2017;10(4):580–600.
44. American Telemedicine Association guidelines. Available at: https://www.americantelemed.org/search?executeSearch=true&SearchTerm=guidelines&l=1. Accessed August 17, 2017.

45. Heam M, Hyeladzira G, Raymond O. Critical appraisal of published systematic reviews assessing the cost-effectiveness of telemedicine studies. Telemed J E Health 2014;29(7):609–18.
46. Bashshur RL, Shannon GW, Bashshur N, et al. The empirical evidence for telemedicine interventions in mental disorders. Telemed J E Health 2016;22(2): 87–113.
47. Bashshur RL, Shannon GW, Smith BR, et al. The empirical evidence for the telemedicine intervention in diabetes management. Telemed J E Health 2015;21(5): 321–54.
48. Bashshur RL, Shannon GW, Tejasvi T, et al. The empirical foundations of teledermatology: a review of the research evidence. Telemed J E Health 2015;21(12): 953–79.
49. Bashshur RL, Krupinski EA, Thrall JH, et al. The empirical foundations of teleradiology and related applications: a review of the evidence. Telemed J E Health 2016;22(11):868–98.
50. Bashshur RL, Krupinski EA, Weinstein RS, et al. The empirical foundations of telepathology: evidence of feasibility and intermediate effects. Telemed J E Health 2017;23(3):155–91.

Clinical Skills Assessment in the Twenty-First Century

Andrew Elder, BSc, MBCHB, FRCP, FRCPSG, FRCP(Edin)

KEYWORDS

- Medical education • Clinical skills • Assessment • Physical examination

KEY POINTS

- Assessment drives learning and remains fundamental to the acquisition of competence.
- The purpose of the assessment shapes the format chosen.
- Uncertainty exists regarding the best balance between summative (pass-fail) and formative (developmental) assessments in driving the acquisition of clinical skills.
- US GME is unusual, in international terms, in restricting assessment of clinical skills to formative workplace-based settings.

INTRODUCTION

Clinical skills remain fundamental to the practice of medicine and form a core component of the professional identity of the physician. However, evidence exists to suggest that the practice of some clinical skills is declining, particularly in the United States.[1] A decline in practice of any skill can lead to a decline in its teaching and assessment, with further decline in practice as a result. Consequently, assessment not only drives learning of clinical skills, but their practice. This article summarizes contemporary approaches to clinical skills assessment that, if more widely adopted, could support the maintenance and reinvigoration of bedside clinical skills.

WHAT ARE CLINICAL SKILLS?

Clinical skills are typically regarded as the combination of:

- The gathering of clinical information by talk and touch (the history and physical examination)
- The interpretation and application of information gathered by these processes (diagnostic reasoning and clinical thinking)

Disclosure Statement: None.
Department of Acute Medicine for Older People, Edinburgh Medical School, Western General Hospital, Crewe Road, Edinburgh EH42XU, UK
E-mail address: atelder@gmail.com

Med Clin N Am 102 (2018) 545–558
https://doi.org/10.1016/j.mcna.2017.12.014
0025-7125/18/Crown Copyright © 2017 Published by Elsevier Inc. All rights reserved.

- The communication of information to patients and family (counseling) and to colleagues
- The performance of practical procedures

The acquisition of clinical skills depends on learning how to perform certain motor skills (procedural knowledge), understanding why one should perform these skills (factual knowledge of basic medical sciences), and applying reasoning to interpret the findings from skills (conditional knowledge).[2] This is shown schematically in **Fig. 1**.

In clinical practice, and in teaching and assessment, it is often difficult to dissociate one clinical skill from others. As such, the teaching and assessment of each often overlaps with that of others, and indeed must do so if validity is to be maximized and professional competence, rather than mere performance of an individual skill, measured. Because the teaching and assessment of practical procedures is usually regarded separately in the educational literature, it is not covered in this article.

WHAT ARE WE TRYING TO ASSESS?

The acquisition of competence, variously defined as the ability to undertake a specific task, or a component of activity that a professional must undertake within a task, is the aim of teaching and learning in medicine. Different assessment methods are suggested for different components of competence,[3] as illustrated in **Fig. 2**.

In this model, assessing "does" is regarded as more authentic, and thus important, than assessing "shows how." This has led to an emphasis on workplace assessments conducted while the learner actually "does" the tasks their role requires them to perform.

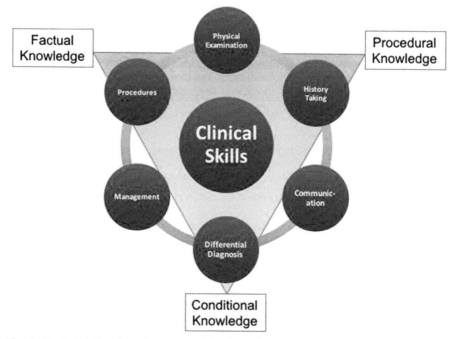

Fig. 1. Clinical skills: what they are and the knowledge that underpins their acquisition. (*Data from* Michels ME, Evans DE, Blok GA. What is a clinical skill? Searching for order in chaos through a modified Delphi process. Med Teach 2012;34(8):e573–81.)

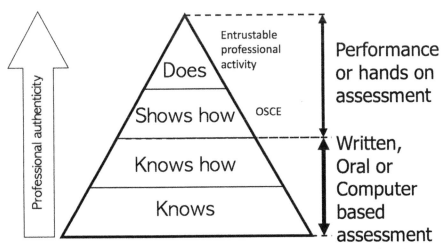

Fig. 2. Components of competence and their matching assessments. OSCE, objective structured clinical examination.

Current thinking promotes Entrustable Professional Activities as a practicable means of ensuring the professional competence of learners.[4] In this method, multiple informing competencies are combined into broader areas of professional activity, and assessment based at the level of the activity rather than the competence. For example, an expected professional activity for an internal medicine resident is the assessment of a new referral in an out-patient clinic. Successful delivery of this activity depends on many competencies, including the ability to take a history, undertake a physical examination, and communicate information to the patient. In basing assessment at the level of the activity, it is assumed that successful performance of the activity means that each informing competency has also been successfully attained.

This model may therefore be best suited to those nearing certification. At other stages of education, greater focus may be required on individual informing competencies; for example, the method of physical examination should be specifically assessed in the prelicensing medical student. Arguably, it should not be assumed that these specific informing competencies will be maintained into graduate medical education (GME); the Entrustable Professional Activities method may incorrectly assume that they are. Suggested differences in focus at different stages of medical education are shown in **Fig. 3**.

WHAT IS THE PURPOSE OF ASSESSMENT?

Assessment has a variety of functions in medical education, some of which are summarized in **Box 1**. The purpose of assessment should dictate the type of assessment chosen.

WHAT FACTORS INFORM THE CHOICE OF ASSESSMENT USED?

A key first step in the design of any assessment is the consideration of its purpose; its form follows its function. That is, an assessment that must primarily be developmental takes one form, and one that must set an objective standard to be attained takes another.

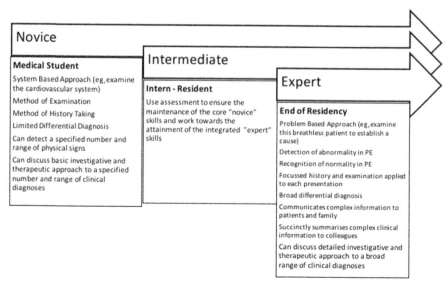

Fig. 3. From novice to expert: shifting the focus of assessment of clinical skills over time. PE, physical examination.

Other considerations must be applied when considering the format of an assessment. Reliability, or reproducibility, is traditionally believed to more important in summative than formative settings. Validity, which may be regarded as how closely the assessment measures what it is intended to measure, is said to be easier to achieve in workplace-based settings. Practicality is an additional factor; assessments using real patients may not be feasible for large cohorts of learners. Other logistic factors also influence choice, such as "What space is available for the assessment? and "How many faculty are willing and able to be involved?" The overall utility of an assessment has been expressed in conceptual form,[5] as shown in **Fig. 4**.

In addition to psychometric and practical characteristics of each assessment method, the educational impact, and, in the opinion of this author, the public message that the assessment provides, should be considered. Specifically, high stakes assessments of clinical skills send a clear signal to the public that these skills are taken seriously by the profession.[6]

Box 1
Some purposes of assessment in medical education

Ensure minimum standards of knowledge or skills

Rank or grade trainees for selection or other purposes

Inform licensing, certification, or other key progression decisions

Provide a forum for direct observation of clinical skills

Provide feedback to the learner on performance of clinical skills

Provide feedback to the teacher on the progression of the learner

Provide feedback to the teacher on the impact of a teaching program

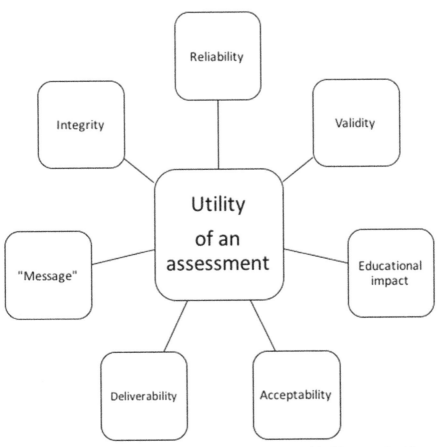

Fig. 4. Factors contributing to the utility of an assessment. (*Modified from* Van Der Vleuten CP. The assessment of professional competence: developments, research and practical implications. Adv Health Sci Educ Theory Pract 1996;1(1):41–67; with permission.)

FORMATIVE AND SUMMATIVE ASSESSMENTS

Assessments *for* learning, or formative assessments, are developmental, with the primary intention of providing feedback to the learner, thus aiding the acquisition of new skills or knowledge. Assessments *of* learning, or summative assessments, are designed to ensure attainment of a specific standard at a specific point in time. The relative advantages and disadvantages of formative workplace-based and high stakes assessments of clinical skills are summarized in **Table 1**.

Development of the learner and the acquisition of competence are critically dependent on direct observation and feedback delivered as close to the learning event as is possible.[7] This, coupled with the view that authenticity of assessment is greatest when the assessment is structured around the performance of a real clinical activity, has given emphasis to workplace assessment in recent years.

However, it has proven difficult to ensure that faculty has the time and expertise to deliver workplace assessments to a sufficient standard and frequency.[8] Some observers also point to the lack of independence of workplace assessors[9] and the

Table 1
Comparative characteristics of formative and summative assessment of clinical skills

Formative: In Workplace	Summative: At Venue Other than Workplace
Easier to give immediate feedback and remediation	Harder to give immediate feedback and remediation
Harder to make pass standard the same across assessment venues	Easier to make pass standard the same across assessment venues
Assessor more likely to know the trainee; can lack impartiality	Assessor does not know the trainee; independent, impartial judgment
Less resource (time and money) intensive	More resource (time and money) intensive
Delivery of the assessment harder to standardize	Delivery of the assessment easier to standardize
Candidate may know patient	Candidate less likely to know patient
Assessor training harder to standardize in multiple venues	Assessor training easier to standardize
Can be difficult to translate formative results or judgments into summative progression or pass fail decisions	Easier to construct an agreed pass/fail standard
Arguably of higher validity (assuming real patients used)	Arguably of lower validity (if in nonclinical setting and using simulated patients)
More difficult to make reliable/reproducible	Easier to make reliable/reproducible
Harder to quality assure	Easier to quality assure
Difficult to derive a rank or grade	Easier to derive rank or grade

increasing complexity of systems that prove challenging for faculty to deliver.[10] Furthermore, although learners appreciate observation and feedback, they may find the experience intimidating if it is to be used to inform their progression. In UK GME, workplace assessments have been retitled "supervised learning events," to minimize the sense that they are in any way summative. In addition, it is always necessary to make progression decisions by some method, and it has proven difficult to translate ratings derived from global workplace assessments of clinical skills into reliable pass/fail classifications or grades.[11]

Given these issues, most GME systems around the world continue to use summative high stakes clinical skills examinations to inform key progression decisions in medicine, such as those relating to licensing and certification, in combination with the information derived from workplace-based assessments.[12] No specific combination of formative and summative methods has been found to be more successful in ensuring the attainment of any specific level of clinical skill. In most educational programs, a variety of assessment methods are used, to maximize the information known about each learner, and triangulate assessment between multiple assessors and complementary methods, within the overall concept of "programmatic assessment."[13]

THE UNITED STATES APPROACH

US GME assessment in internal medicine is unusual in global educational terms, in that assessment of clinical skills after the point of licensing is wholly based on assessments of fundamentally formative style, delivered in the learner's workplace. Summative assessments *the Boards* are restricted to assessments of knowledge, which can assess aspects of clinical thinking, and theoretic knowledge underpinning clinical skills, but clearly cannot assess the actual practice of these skills. This approach contrasts starkly with other GME systems around the world, including in Australia, Canada, Ireland, and the United Kingdom, that require success in a high stakes summative assessment of clinical skills as a mandatory component of progression, and thus certification, in addition to completion of workplace-based assessments.

Critics of high stakes clinical skills examinations point to their potential cost, low validity (particularly if simulation is used), the difficulties of ensuring sufficient interrater reliability to support a pass/fail decision, and learner stress as justifications for their exclusion from assessment systems. However, the educational impact of these examinations on learners and faculty is substantial,[6] and the consequences of their absence from an assessment system must be taken into as much consideration as would the absence of high stakes assessments of knowledge.

SOME SPECIFIC WORKPLACE ASSESSMENTS OF CLINICAL SKILLS
Mini-CEX

The mini-CEX[14] evolved from the CEX, which was promoted as an alternative to a summative clinical skills examination when the American Board of Internal Medicine dropped an oral clinical skills examination in 1972. The CEX was time consuming, and suffered from the same problems as similar assessments delivered in a summative setting, with case specificity and assessor inconsistency foremost. The mini-CEX is shorter (15–20 minutes) and theoretically permits sampling of a wider range of skills across a range of encounters, by different faculty members. Time for feedback is increased, construct and criterion validity high, and derived judgements more reliable.[15]

Case-Based Discussion

This is a form of chart-stimulated oral discussion, which is used to assess diagnostic reasoning and management planning, but does not typically involve direct observation of the learner interacting with the patient. Broader professional bedside attributes, such as behavior in teams and professional attitude, may be assessed by peer or colleague review in "Multi-source Feedback" but are beyond the scope of this article.

SUMMATIVE ASSESSMENTS OF CLINICAL SKILLS
Traditional Models

Assessments of bedside clinical skills should ideally assess information gathering, synthesis, analysis and application of gathered information, and its communication. Traditional summative clinical skills examinations attempted to cover these domains in the "short case–long case–viva" model.

The short cases
In this format, candidates are asked to examine one part of the patient (eg, the hands or facies) to describe what they see or find and suggest the cause, directly observed and in discussion with one or two examiners. A short introductory statement is provided, typically in the form of a one line history: "This patient has painful hands." No communication with the patient is typically permitted.

The ability to elicit and interpret signs, diagnostic reasoning, and clinical thinking is assessed and, given the brevity of each encounter, sampling across different organ systems or conditions can occur. However, some of what is assessed is more consistently assessed with photographic or video material. Validity is clearly impaired if the candidate is not allowed to take a history, and detailed guidance may be necessary to standardize examiner-candidate interaction, and questions asked. Despite these limitations, this model is still used in many assessment settings.

The long case

The candidate spends up to an hour with a patient, typically unobserved. They then present the case to one or more examiners, and may discuss aspects of differential diagnosis, and clinical thinking relating to investigation and management. The candidate may be taken back to the bedside to demonstrate physical signs. This format has good face validity and contains elements of the "case-based discussion" or chart stimulated recall formats now used in workplace assessments. However, critics of its use in a summative setting point to the fact that style of communication, attitudes and behaviors with the patient, and method of physical examination are not directly observed and cannot be assessed. Standardization of the examiner-candidate interaction is also seen as a limitation, as is standardization of the clinical content, because different patients may present markedly different challenges.

The Objective Structured Long Examination Record was introduced as a means of attempting to standardize the long case assessment and improve its objectivity, validity, and reliability. The 10-point checklist helped examiners to structure the areas of assessment and was conceptually important, but gained little practical support and is not now widely used.[16]

The viva

The traditional viva or oral examination is a means of assessing applied clinical knowledge, particularly diagnostic reasoning, knowledge of methods of investigation, or guidelines for treatment. Critics cite inconsistency in the examiner-candidate interaction, the long testing time required to produce adequate reliability, and the fact that much of what is assessed is assessed more effectively in written examination settings, as justifications for exclusion from assessment programs. Despite this, viva examinations persist in many international medical assessment settings.

Newer Models

Newer models of summative clinical skills assessment attempt to find a balance between validity, reliability, and practicality.[12] No model is perfect, and inclusion of a summative skills examination in an assessment system is inherently associated with acceptance of a compromise between these different elements.

Reliability is enhanced by standardization of content and interaction between candidate and examiner. Emphasis is placed on sampling across and between skills and across multiple diseases or presentations in a series of encounters. Direct observation of candidate-patient interactions, usually by an expert clinician examiner, is regarded as important. Most formats retain some examiner-candidate interaction, but in some, most notably the USMLE Clinical Skills Step 2 examination, where the simulated patient also takes the role of examiner, there is no interaction other than that demanded by the simulated clinical encounter.

Assessment theory also suggests that interactions between candidate and patient should be as standardized as possible. In examinations with many candidates the consequence of this thinking is that standardized or simulated patients are used.

Although this may not affect the assessment of method of physical examination, it greatly limits the assessment of the ability to elicit abnormal physical signs and is believed to reduce validity.

The objective structured clinical examination

The Objective Structured Clinical Examination[17] was developed as an alternative to traditional models of clinical examinations and typically takes the form of a circuit of stations, each of one or more clinical encounter or linked clinical task (eg, writing a prescription for a patient assessed in the previous encounter), some of which is observed by at least one examiner, who is usually a more senior clinician.

Uncertainty and debate persist about the optimal number of stations, the length of the stations, the number of examiners, whether all tasks are observed, and relative benefits of real and simulated patients.[18] In practice, these psychometric and academic considerations must be balanced against the resources available (ie, the availability of time, space, faculty to act as examiners, and patients to participate).

Key considerations in the construction of a summative clinical skills examination are summarized in **Box 2**.

Box 2
Some factors to consider in the design of a summative assessment of clinical skills

Will it use real or simulated patients/mannequins, or both?

Will the candidate-patient interaction be observed or unobserved?

If observed, will the examiner be a clinician or a trained lay person, or both, and how many examiners will there be?

What interaction between candidates and examiners will be permitted?

Will marking be based on an itemized checklist or global rating scale?

What domains of performance will be defined and assessed?

Will the pass standard permit compensation between different domains, or must each be passed separately?

Will clinical challenges be based on a system (eg, cardiovascular) or a symptom or presentation?

What level of interaction between the patient and candidate is permitted (physical examination stations)

How many stations/encounters can be accommodated, and are necessary?

How long will each encounter be?

Will some encounters include data or image interpretation, with or without a patient present?

How will the degree of difficulty of each encounter be graded and/or compared and/or standardized?

Will there be any sequential or "linked" encounters, with tasks that follow from an interaction at a previous encounter?

Will some encounters assess specific clinical skills only (eg, physical examination) or will all attempt to integrate all clinical skills?

How will the pass standard be set?

How will feedback be provided to candidates? (pass/fail classification only: Score and Rank: Examiner comments)

SPECIFIC SUMMATIVE CLINICAL SKILLS EXAMINATIONS OF INTEREST
USMLE Step 2 Clinical Skills

The USMLE Step 2 CS examination[19] is the largest graduation or licensing level examination in the world, with more than 30,000 candidates per annum examined in five centers. It is highly standardized, and of good published reliability, but critics point to the fact that interactions are not observed, that assessment of the interaction is by a trained simulated patient rather than a clinician expert, that no real patients and thus real physical signs can be included, that feedback is limited, and that costs for candidates are high. A noncompensatory three-domain marking structure is used, in which performance is assessed in the Integrated Clinical Encounter, Spoken English Proficiency, and Communication and Interpersonal Skills, with a separate pass standard required in each.

Running in parallel with final examinations in US medical schools, its prime purpose is to ensure, with a high degree of reliability, that a minimum standard of clinical practice is attained by US and international medical graduates. In achieving that aim, it remains the prime example of a successful, high-volume, summative clinical skills examination.

It is noteworthy that this is the last summative assessment of bedside clinical skills that most practitioners of internal medicine in the United States undergo. For some, it may even be the last time that the basic clinical skills of physical examination and history taking are ever directly observed, albeit by a trained simulated patient, rather than a faculty member or other expert clinician examiner.

The MRCP(UK) Practical Assessment of Clinical Examination Skills Examination

The Practical Assessment of Clinical Examination Skills (PACES)[20] is the largest summative international GME examination of clinical skills in the world, sat by around 5000 doctors annually. It is the third part of the MRCP(UK) Diploma examination, the first two parts being knowledge-based examinations in single best answer, best of five options format, with content and standard like that of the American Board of Internal Medicine Certification examinations. Successful completion is mandatory for certification in internal medicine.

PACES provides a portable objective structured clinical examination–based model in which candidates rotate around five stations each of 20 minutes, each station comprised of one to two patient encounters (**Fig. 5**).

A total of eight patients are seen in these encounters, of which a minimum of four are real patients with real physical findings. All candidate-patient interactions are directly observed by two examiners, such that a total of 10 examiners have observed and assessed the candidates over the duration of the examination. Examiners independently mark seven defined domains of clinical skills (**Table 2**).[21]

Candidates are assessed using a structured domain-based marking system, which is a compromise between an itemized checklist and global rating scale, these two methods having attracted considerable academic interest.[22,23] Limited interaction between one of the two examiners and the candidate occurs at each encounter, but most of the assessment is based on observation of the candidates. Because real patients participate, a specific method of minimizing variation between examiner assessment is used, entitled calibration. In this process, pairs of examiners personally evaluate the clinical findings of each patient before the examination starts, to establish the findings; grade their difficulty; and agree what methods, findings, and applied knowledge are required to justify the award of a satisfactory grade for those domains.

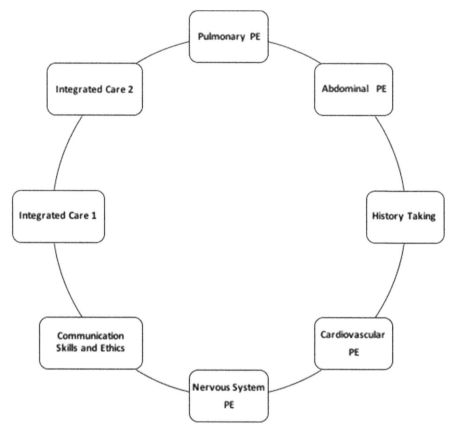

Fig. 5. The MRCP(UK) Paces Carousel. (*Adapted from* Elder A, McManus C, McAlpine L, et al. What skills are tested in the New PACES Examination? Ann Acad Med Singapore 2011;40(3):120; with permission.)

The examination is resource and time intensive; only five candidates are assessed by 10 examiners, using up to six real and four simulated patients, over 125 minutes. Reliability, which is difficult to calculate in an examination with eight separate pass standards, meets the UK medical regulator, the General Medical Council, requirement for a high stakes examination. PACES includes encounters that integrate history and physical examination and in doing so with real patients enhances validity, but at the expense of standardization and hence reliability.

The Place of Simulation

Practical considerations relating to the number of candidates requiring assessment have led to widespread use of surrogates and actors as simulated patients, typically performing to a strictly defined script, in many examinations.[24] Simulation of this sort improves standardization of content, but may compromise validity, particularly if mannequins or computer-based avatars are used as representations of patients. This increase of the use of simulation, to aid the logistics of delivery and improve standardization, should not be interpreted as overall evidence of superiority over examinations in which clinical content is based on real patients, and it remains to be seen

Table 2
Seven domains of clinical skills assessed in the MRCP(UK) PACES examination

	Clinical Skill	Skill Descriptor
A	Physical examination	Demonstrate correct, thorough, systematic (or focused in Station 5 encounters), appropriate, fluent, and professional technique of physical examination.
B	Identifying physical signs	Identify physical signs that are present correctly, and not find physical signs that are not present.
C	Clinical communication	Elicit a clinical history relevant to the patient's complaints, in a systematic, thorough (or focused in Station 5 encounters), fluent, and professional manner. Explain relevant clinical information in an accurate, clear, structured, comprehensive, fluent, and professional manner.
D	Differential diagnosis	Create a sensible differential diagnosis for a patient that the candidate has personally clinically assessed.
E	Clinical judgment	Select or negotiate a sensible and appropriate management plan for a patient, relative, or clinical situation. Select appropriate investigations or treatments for a patient that the candidate has personally clinically assessed. Apply clinical knowledge, including knowledge of law and ethics, to the case.
F	Managing patients' concerns	Seek, detect, acknowledge, and address patients' or relatives' concerns. Listen to a patient or relative, confirm their understanding of the matter under discussion, and demonstrate empathy.
G	Maintaining patient welfare	Treat a patient or relative respectfully and sensitively and in a manner that ensures their comfort, safety, and dignity.

Adapted from Elder A, McManus C, McAlpine L, et al. What skills are tested in the New PACES Examination? Ann Acad Med Singapore 2011;40(3):121; with permission.

whether the apparent benefits of simulation translate into improved core bedside clinical skills, and overall clinical competence, when practiced on real patients.[25]

SUMMARY AND FUTURE CONSIDERATIONS

The quality of assessment of clinical skills influences the quality of their practice, and vice versa. If practice is to be sustained or reinvigorated, frequent, structured assessment must occur, particularly in GME. Although psychometric considerations relating to reliability and standardization cannot be entirely overlooked, they should not become an absolute barrier to the occurrence of some form of assessment, because the educational impact of the absence of any assessment of clinical skills is likely to be significant. At the GME level, direct observation by faculty, with clinical encounters that include real patients with real physical findings, is highly preferable.[26] Whether the assessment is primarily summative or formative is of secondary importance, and hybrid models should be considered. In short, the most important thing about a clinical skills assessment is that it happens—everything else is detail.

REFERENCES

1. Vukanovic-Criley JM, Criley S, Warde CM, et al. Competency cardiac examination skills in medical students, trainees, physicians and faculty: a multicenter study. Arch Intern Med 2006;166:610–6.

2. Michels ME, Evans DE, Blok GA. What is a clinical skill? Searching for order in chaos through a modified Delphi process. Med Teach 2012;34(8):e573–81.

3. Miller GE. The assessment of clinical skills/competence/performance. Acad Med 1990;65:S63–7.

4. Ten Cate O. Nuts and bolts of entrustable professional activities. J Grad Med Educ 2013;5(1):157–8.

5. van der Vleuten CP. The assessment of professional competence: developments, research and practical implications. Adv Health Sci Educ Theory Pract 1996;1(1): 41–67.

6. Elder AT. In praise of clinical examinations (Editorial). Clin Med 2014;14(5):460–1.

7. Holmboe ES. Faculty and the observation of trainees' clinical skills: problems and opportunities. Acad Med 2004;79(1):16–22.

8. Chaudhry SI, Holmboe E, Beasley BW. The state of evaluation in internal medicine residency. J Gen Intern Med 2008;23(7):1010–5.

9. Cavalcanti RB, Detsky AS. The education and training of future physicians: why coaches can't be judges. JAMA 2011;306(9):993–4.

10. Witteles RM, Verghese A. Accreditation council for graduate medical education (ACGME) milestones—time for a revolt? JAMA Intern Med 2016;176(11): 1599–600.

11. Jackson JL, Kay C, Frank M. The validity and reliability of attending evaluations of medicine residents. SAGE Open Med 2015;3. 2050312115589648.

12. Wass V, Van der Vleuten C, Shatzer J, et al. Assessment of clinical competence. Lancet 2001;357(9260):945–9.

13. van der Vleuten CP, Schuwirth LW, Driessen EW, et al. A model for programmatic assessment fit for purpose. Med Teach 2012;34(3):205–14.

14. Norcini JJ, Blank LL, Duffy FD, et al. The mini-CEX: a method for assessing clinical skills. Ann Intern Med 2003;138(6):476–81.

15. Al Ansari A, Ali SKK, Donnon T. The construct and criterion validity of the mini-CEX: a meta-analysis of the published research. Acad Med 2013;88(3): 413–20.

16. Gleeson F. AMEE medical education guide no 9: assessment of clinical competence using the objective structured long examination record (OSLER). Med Teach 1997;19:7–14.

17. Harden RM, Gleeson FA. Assessment of clinical competence using an objective structured clinical examination (OSCE). Med Education 1979;13(1):39–54.

18. Turner JL, Dankoski ME. Objective structured clinical exams: a critical review. Fam Med 2008;40(8):574–8.

19. Available at: http://www.usmle.org/step-2-cs/. Accessed August 1, 2017.

20. Available at: https://www.mrcpuk.org/mrcpuk-examinations/paces. Accessed August 1, 2017.

21. Elder AT, McManus IC, McAlpine LG, et al. What skills are tested in the new PACES examination? Ann Acad Med Singapore 2011;40:119–25.

22. Allen R, Heard S, Savidge M. Global ratings versus checklist scoring in an OSCE. Acad Med 1998;73:597–8.

23. Ilgen JS, Ma IW, Hatala R, et al. A systematic review of validity evidence for checklists versus global rating scales in simulation-based assessment. Med Education 2015;49(2):161–73.

24. Dillon GF, Boulet JR, Hawkins RE, et al. Simulations in the United States Medical Licensing Examination (USMLE). Qual Saf Health Care 2004;13(Suppl 1): i41–5.

25. Ryall T, Judd BK, Gordon CJ. Simulation-based assessments in health professional education: a systematic review. J Multidiscip Healthc 2016;9:69–82.

26. Fromme HB, Karani R, Downing SM. Direct observation in medical education: a review of the literature and evidence for validity. Mt Sinai J Med 2009;76(4): 365–71.

Digital Tools to Enhance Clinical Reasoning

Reza Manesh, MD[a],*, Gurpreet Dhaliwal, MD[b,c]

KEYWORDS

- Clinical reasoning • Diagnostic skills • Virtual patients • Clinical problem-solving

KEY POINTS

- Physicians can improve their diagnostic accuracy by adopting a simulation-based approach to reading published cases.
- Virtual patients are computer-based programs that foster learning through simulation of real-life case scenarios.
- The move from static formats to electronic platforms increases the accessibility of cases and makes learning more active and durable.

INTRODUCTION

A core component of providing excellent patient care is analyzing and synthesizing clinical data to arrive at the correct diagnosis. Despite the increasing demands placed on clinicians, physicians owe it to their patients to constantly seek ways to improve their diagnostic accuracy. Methods to enhance knowledge and improve clinical reasoning skills that underpin diagnostic excellence are point-of-care learning, feedback, simulation, and deliberate practice.[1]

Technology does not provide a shortcut to clinical excellence but it does lower the barrier to building knowledge and developing reasoning skills that lead to outstanding clinical performance (**Table 1**). This article highlights online resources that can increase the number of cases a clinician can experience and learn from.

Disclosure Statement: Dr R. Manesh is supported by the Jeremiah A. Barondess Fellowship in the Clinical Transaction of the New York Academy of Medicine, in collaboration with the Accreditation Council for Graduate Medical Education (ACGME). Dr R. Manesh receives an honorarium from the Human Diagnosis Project for serving as Global Morning Report supervising editor. Dr G. Dhaliwal reports receiving honoraria from ISMIE Mutual Insurance Company and Physicians' Reciprocal Insurers.

[a] Department of Internal Medicine, Johns Hopkins Hospital, Johns Hopkins University School of Medicine, 600 North Wolfe Street, Meyer 8-34D, Baltimore, MD 21287, USA; [b] Department of Medicine, University of California San Francisco, San Francisco, CA, USA; [c] Medical Service, San Francisco VA Medical Center, 4150 Clement Street, San Francisco, CA 94121, USA
* Corresponding author.
E-mail address: rsedigh1@jhmi.edu

Med Clin N Am 102 (2018) 559–565
https://doi.org/10.1016/j.mcna.2017.12.015
0025-7125/18/© 2017 Elsevier Inc. All rights reserved.

Table 1		
Enhancing clinical reasoning through technology		
Task	**Purpose**	**Examples**
Build general knowledge	Augment knowledge for unspecified future encounters	• Journal table of contents email alerts • Journal & FOAM podcasts • Journal & FOAM Twitter accounts
Build case-specific knowledge	Augment knowledge in real time for current encounters	• UpToDate • Google • PubMed
Decision support	Augment decision making in real time for current encounters	• Isabel • VisualDx • DxPlain
Feedback	Learn from patient outcomes	• Electronic medical record • Asynchronous electronic communication with other clinicians
Simulation	Practice with additional cases	• *New England Journal of Medicine* Interactive Cases • *Journal of General Internal Medicine* Exercises in Clinical Reasoning • Human Diagnosis Project

Abbreviation: FOAM, free open access medical education.

WHY CASES?

Professionals who wish to improve their knowledge and performance seek opportunities to practice their relevant skill. Experts in chess, the military, and aviation practice their craft through self-created or externally imposed simulations. Medicine has embraced simulation for psyhomotor skills like laparoscopic surgery but not for cognitive skills.

Published cases simulate the diagnostic journey of the treating clinicians. The tight coupling of clinical problems and their solutions affords readers the opportunity to efficiently upgrade their illness scripts (structured knowledge of a specific disease) and schemas (structured frameworks for common problems). The more times clinicians practice accessing and applying those knowledge structures, the better their approach will be to future patient-cases. Although the final diagnosis at the end of published cases is sometimes rare, it is the journey that provides lessons for everyday patient encounters (eg, approach to dyspnea, anemia, or renal injury).[2]

Virtual patients (VPs) are computer-based programs that foster learning through simulation of real-life case scenarios.[3] Well-designed VPs allow users to practice decisions and learn from feedback. VPs also integrate distractors such as misleading test results and extraneous information that mimic authentic clinical environments. Learning theory and education reviews propose that the greatest pedagogical value of VPs is the enhancement of clinical reasoning skills.[4] VPs aim to transform abstract knowledge into tacit knowledge through active problem solving.

THE CLINICAL PROBLEM-SOLVING FORMAT CASE

Medical journals (such as the *New England Journal of Medicine, Journal of Hospital Medicine,* and *Journal of General Internal Medicine*) publish cases in the clinical problem-solving format. In these series, a case is presented in a step-wise fashion where each portion of the case chronology (eg, history of illness or laboratory test results) is followed by an expert's analysis. The following approach can enhance the challenge (and learning) that comes from reading a clinical problem-solving case:

- Avoid the title of the case, as it often hints at the final diagnosis.
- Do not look ahead at any images, as it might bias your clinical reasoning (eg, an early glance at a pathology slide may limit the diagnostic possibilities you contend with).
- After analyzing one section of case data, skip the expert's discussion, and move on to the next section; often the expert suggests or arrives at the diagnosis early in the case, which artificially influences your thinking in subsequent sections.
- Stop after each section and write down your assessment: How are you framing the case? What is your working diagnosis? What would be your next steps?
- Commit to a final diagnosis before it is revealed at the end of the case; getting feedback on your decisions is the only way to refine your judgment.
- Return to the beginning of the case and compare your sequential assessments with the expert's evolving thinking during the case.
- Read the commentary that follows the case and create or refine your illness scripts and schemas for the relevant diseases and problems, respectively.

Reading cases in this way recreates the struggle of the treating clinicians and allows the reader to compare how they would handle the situation against the decisions of the treating clinicians and expert discussant. This approach fortifies the reader's knowledge structures (illness scripts), approaches to problems (schemas), and ability to discern the most important elements of a complex case (problem representation).

When approached in this way, print-based cases are effective forms of clinical reasoning practice. Electronic platforms can make this exercise more efficient and more engaging. The following sections outline 3 formats of online cases (**Table 2**). The first 2 feature traditional print media cases that are enhanced by online presentations. The third is exclusively online. All of the featured resources are free.

Journal of General Internal Medicine: Exercises in Clinical Reasoning

The Exercises in Clinical Reasoning (ECR) series of the *Journal of General Internal Medicine* (*JGIM*) presents a challenging case with an in-depth focus on the clinician's cognitive strategies.[5] By analyzing the clinician's thought process, core concepts and strategies in clinical reasoning are highlighted.

Technology-enhanced learning
A select number of published ECR cases are grouped into an online toolbox with extra features to enhance understanding of the underlying clinical reasoning theme.[6] Each concept is highlighted on a Web page and includes a link to the ECR case, an introductory document that highlights the reasoning concept's application in daily practice, and a slide deck of the case.

Example The ECR case, "A 22-Year-Old Woman with Abdominal Pain"[7], defines and examines the illness scripts concept through a case of abdominal pain. The slides provide the reader with a visual representation of the components of an illness script for a disease: pathophysiology, epidemiology, time course, symptoms and signs, diagnostics, and treatment. The case begins with a 22-year-old woman with 2 days of abdominal pain. The slide deck invites the reader to elaborate the illness scripts of leading diagnoses. The reader later has the opportunity to review illness scripts for 4

Table 2
Online case-based simulations

Resource	Typical Time per Case	Distinguishing Features	Similar Digital Resources
Journal of General Internal Medicine Exercises in Clinical Reasoning	30–60 min	• Teacher's guide • Practice applying clinical reasoning concepts	
New England Journal of Medicine Interactive Medical Cases	30–60 min	• Multimedia learning modules • Performance score compared with other users	• i-Human Patients • MedU • *The Lancet* Interactive Ground Round series • *Annals of Internal Medicine* Virtual Patients
Human Diagnosis Project	5–10 min	• Comparison with differential diagnosis of other users • Performance score compared with other users	• QuantiaMD • The JN (*JAMA* Network) Challenge

candidate diseases by clicking on hyperlinks for Crohn's disease, acute mesenteric ischemia, herpes zoster, and adrenal insufficiency. Before the final diagnosis is revealed, the presentation calls on the reader to compare and contrast the illness scripts of the candidate diagnoses.

Technology-enhanced teaching

The online ECRs feature a teaching guide with each slide deck. As the case unfolds, the educator can use strategies outlined in the teacher's notes to interact with trainees, such as soliciting the components of an illness script for a common diagnosis. Selected slides have questions that prompt the group to reflect on the clinical reasoning process (metacognition).

Summary

The *JGIM* ECR series simultaneously enhances knowledge of medical and clinical reasoning concepts. Online ECRs allow readers to examine clinical reasoning concepts and teach those concepts to trainees and colleagues.

The New England Journal of Medicine Interactive Medical Case Series

The *New England Journal of Medicine* (*NEJM*) Clinical Problem-Solving (CPS) series presents case information in stages to an experienced clinician who reveals their sequential thinking. In 2009, the *NEJM* launched the Interactive Medical Case (IMC) series, which is a collection of online cases (virtual patients) that follow the CPS format.[8] Some cases appear in the print journal as a CPS and online as an IMC; other cases are only presented as an IMC.

Technology-enhanced learning

The *NEJM* Interactive Medical Case utilizes interactive learning features including multiple choice questions (MCQ), matching exercises, and identification tasks.[9] After each challenge, a detailed answer is provided in conjunction with a multimedia presentation. After completing a case, the learner receives an overall score that compares their performance with the worldwide readership.

Example "Dissecting a Case of Abdominal Pain" starts with a 43-year-old man with acute, severe abdominal pain.[10] This opening is followed by an animated physical examination that promotes interpretation and incorporation of key findings (eg, left upper quadrant tenderness) into the reader's working assessment. The first interactive test of knowledge prompts the user to identify 4 conditions that cause acute left upper quadrant pain. A detailed explanation follows each MCQ providing justification (and references) for the correct choice and analysis of the incorrect options. For example, after a splenic infarct is revealed, a module highlights the anatomy and function of the spleen using pathology images.

Technology-enhanced teaching
By projecting the IMC onto a screen and directly teaching from the *NEJM* website, a teacher can lead a group session focused on solving the case. At the predetermined breaks, the teacher can have trainees address the interactive challenge exercises and review the learning elements from the multimedia content.

Summary
The *NEJM* IMCs are professional-grade virtual patients. The interactive elements facilitate decision-making practice and learning about common conditions and relevant pathophysiology through spaced challenges and multimedia teaching content.

The Human Diagnosis Project

The Human Diagnosis Project is an online system that allows physicians to upload and solve cases shared by clinicians worldwide.[11]

Technology-enhanced learning
The Global Morning Report (GMR) series highlights one case per day for the entire community. It takes approximately 5 minutes to solve the GMR case on an electronic device and an additional 3 minutes to review the teaching points. As a patient's case is presented in stages, the system prompts users to enter their leading diagnoses at each step.

An accuracy score reflects how high the correct diagnosis was ranked in the user's final differential diagnosis. An efficiency score reflects the number of clinical data points the user needed before she first included the correct diagnosis in her differential diagnosis. The program also provides users with percentile rankings (compared to all users) in accuracy and efficiency on all cases they analyzed over the previous 14 days.

Example GMR case 192 begins with a 58-year-old woman who presents with confusion and an image of a nonblanching bilateral lower extremity erythematous rash.[12] Users are prompted to enter their early diagnostic considerations (eg, thrombocytopenia, disseminated intravascular coagulation). In the next section, fever and generalized arthralgia are disclosed, prompting users to revise their differential diagnosis (eg, infective endocarditis, Henoch-Schonlein purpura). Then the patient's history of mitral valve prolapse is revealed, which might lead the user to prioritize infective endocarditis. The final 2 findings are a histopathologic image of leukocytoclastic vasculitis and a description of a brain computed tomography revealing age-indeterminate infarcts. At this stage, clinicians must submit their final ranked differential diagnosis. The users then receive a performance score, teaching points, and a listing of diagnoses with their frequencies entered by the community.

Technology-enhanced teaching
The Human Diagnosis Project allows educators to engage multiple trainees simultaneously in the same case. Members of the group (eg, on a small medical team) revise

their differential diagnosis on their devices as each piece of data is revealed. The thinking of the different learners at each stage of the case can be compared and contrasted in a group discussion. The exercise concludes by reviewing the teaching points.

Summary
The Human Diagnosis Project is an efficient way for clinicians to practice their diagnostic skills and compare their performance to their peers. The short time requirement and phone-based application lowers time and accessibility barriers to case-based practice.

SUMMARY

The clinical encounter remains the cornerstone of clinical reasoning growth for all physicians. But the skill level that practitioners achieve from daily experience alone is insufficient. Estimates that 10% to 15% of all clinical encounters have diagnostic errors[13] reminds us that every clinician—whether newly minted or seasoned—has an obligation to continually refine their ability to collect, analyze, and synthesize clinical data. Case-based simulations can improve reasoning skills by increasing the number of episodes of practice that are tightly coupled with feedback. If a day on the front lines diagnosing and treating patients is akin to a cognitive workout, then analyzing additional digital cases is like getting in a few more "reps" at the end of the day.

The move from static (print) formats to digital platforms increases the accessibility of cases and makes the learning more active and durable. This article outlined digital resources that transform the clinician from a passive reader to the front-line physician. The clinician who takes advantage of these resources can increase their experience and their expertise.

REFERENCES

1. Dhaliwal G. Lifelong learning in clinical reasoning. In: Trowbridge RL Jr, Rencic JJ, Durning SJ, editors. Teaching clinical reasoning. Philadelphia: American College of Physicians; 2015. p. 191–204.
2. Peile E. More to be learnt from the discussion than the diagnosis. BMJ 2003; 326(7399):1136.
3. Posel N, Mcgee JB, Fleiszer DM. Twelve tips to support the development of clinical reasoning skills using virtual patient cases. Med Teach 2015;37(9):813–8.
4. Cook DA, Triola MM. Virtual patients: a critical literature review and proposed next steps. Med Educ 2009;43(4):303–11.
5. Henderson M, Keenan C, Kohlwes J, et al. Introducing exercises in clinical reasoning. J Gen Intern Med 2010;25(1):9.
6. Kohlwes J, Connor D, Manesh R. Introduction to exercises in clinical reasoning. In: JGIM web only. Available at: http://www.sgim.org/web-only/clinical-reasoning-exercises. Accessed July 29, 2017.
7. Geha R, Connor D, Kohlwes J, et al. Illness scripts overview. In: JGIM web only. Available at: http://www.sgim.org/web-only/clinical-reasoning-exercises/illness-scripts-overview. Accessed July 29, 2017.
8. McMahon GT, Solomon CG, Ross JJ, et al. Interactive medical cases—a new journal feature. NEJM 2009;361:1113.
9. The New England Journal of Medicine interactive medical cases. Available at: http://www.nejm.org/multimedia/interactive-medical-case. Accessed July 29, 2017.

10. Casey J, Vaidya A, Frank N, et al. In: The new england journal of medicine interactive medical cases. Available at: http://www.nejm.org/doi/full/10.1056/NEJMimc1516704. Accessed July 29, 2017.
11. The Human Diagnosis Project. Available at: https://www.humandx.org/. Accessed July 29, 2017.
12. Hwang J. Global morning report 192. In: The human diagnosis project. Available at: https://www.humandx.org/o/e5bc7iwo5633tzt1p7mrmurz9/solve?s=MR. Accessed July 29, 2017.
13. National Academies of Sciences, Engineering, and Medicine. Improving diagnosis in health care. Washington, DC: The National Academies Press; 2015.

Printed and bound by CPI Group (UK) Ltd, Croydon, CR0 4YY

07/10/2024

01040503-0011